ACL Made Simple

Springer Science+Business Media, LLC

Don Johnson, MD

Carleton University and University of Ottawa, Ottawa, Ontario, Canada

ACL Made Simple

With 163 Illustrations

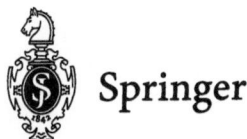

Springer

Don Johnson, MD
Carleton University and University of Ottawa
Ottawa, Ontario, K1S 5B6
Canada

Additional material to this book can be downloaded from http://extras.springer.com

Library of Congress Cataloging-in-Publication Data
Johnson, Don
    ACL made simple / Don Johnson.
      p. cm
    Includes bibliographical references and index.
    ISBN 978-1-4757-8105-2   ISBN 978-0-387-21594-5 (eBook)
    DOI 10.1007/978-0-387-21594-5

    1. Anterior cruciate ligament.   2. Anterior cruciate ligament–Wounds and
injuries–Prevention.   3. Ligaments–Wounds and injuries.   4. Sports injuries.   I. Title.
    RD561.J627 2003
    617.1′027–dc21   2003050496

ISBN 978-1-4757-8105-2   Printed on acid-free paper.

© 2004 Springer Science+Business Media New York
Originally published by Springer-Verlag New York, Inc. in 2004
Softcover reprint of the hardcover 1st edition 2004

9 8 7 6 5 4 3 2 1   SPIN 10931349

www.springer-ny.com

Contents

Contents

1
Introduction

During the past decade, the anterior cruciate ligament (ACL) has become a familiar term. Most athletes have heard about it or know someone who has had an injury to the ACL (Fig. 1.1). This book provides comprehensive information about the ACL that will help the caregiver make an informed decision on the best management of any injury.

The ACL is the main stabilizer of the knee for athletic pivotal activities. The first repair of the cruciate ligament was attributed to Hay Groves in 1917. Then, in the 1930s, Ivor Palmer wrote one of the first definitive monographs on the subject, in which he advocated early surgical repair by suturing the ligament. Although primary suture repair was eventually found to have a high failure rate in athletes, Palmer had set the stage for the aggressive surgical approach of Swedish surgeons. The modern phase of treatment began when Jones, Erickson, and Macintosh all advocated reconstruction, rather than repair, of the ACL with the patellar tendon. In the 1980s, the extra-articular reconstructions, as pioneered by Macintosh, were replaced with the intra-articular reconstructions as popularized by Erickson. The patellar tendon graft was the gold standard in the 1980s, but during the 1990s, as a result of improved graft preparation and fixation, the semitendinosus became more popular.

In the 1970s, the torn ACL was considered the beginning of a progressive deterioration of the knee that often ended an athlete's career. Now many athletes routinely return to play as soon as three to four months after an injury and certainly by the next season. The medical profession has gained considerable experience in the surgical treatment of ACL injuries, but has made little impact in the prevention of the injury, especially among downhill skiers.

The operative treatment has evolved from open procedures performed in the hospital with postoperative casting to arthroscopically performed outpatient procedures with early weight bearing and splint immobilization. The pain control has also improved considerably. This

1

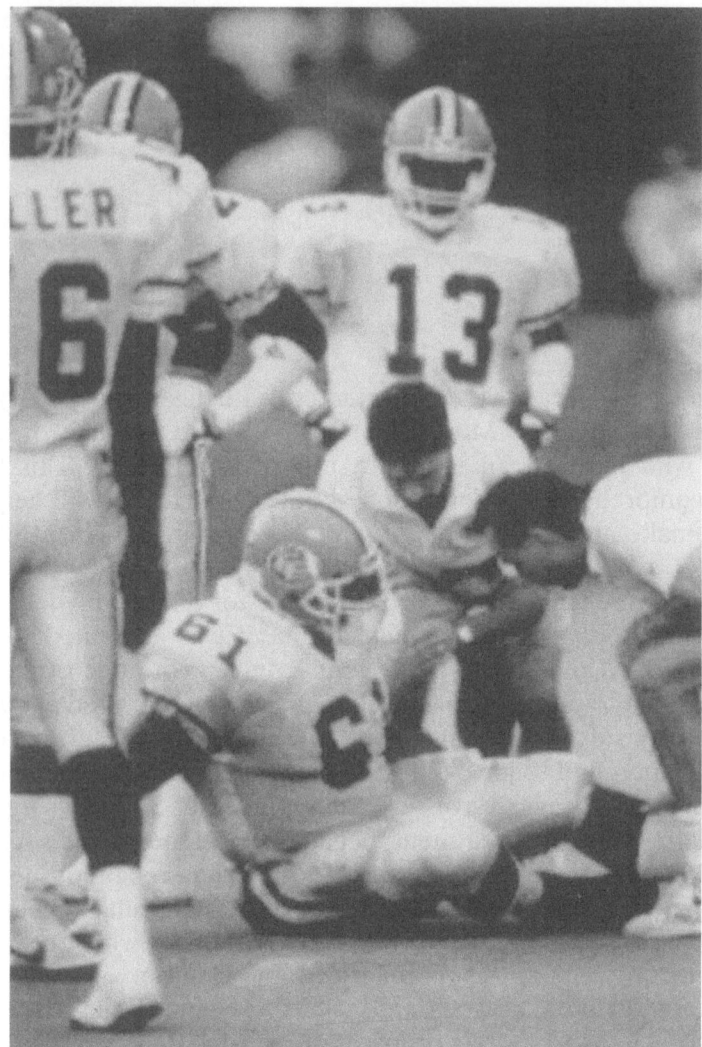

FIGURE 1.1. Injury to the ACL is a common athletic injury.

has lessened the morbidity of the operation and extended the operative option to both the recreational and older athlete.

With the increase in sports participation by the baby boomer generation, injury to the ACL has become one of the most common athletic injuries.

Basic Science

Anatomy

The ACL is composed of two separate bundles, the anteromedial and the posterolateral. The intra-articular length of the ligament is between 28 and 31 mm. The attachment sites on the tibia and femur have a fairly small isometric center (Fig. 1.2).

The ACL and posterior cruciate ligament (PCL) are closely intertwined and are called the "central pivot." An injury to either ligament disrupts the function of the joint and may lead to late degenerative arthritis. The relationship between the ACL and the PCL is shown on the video on the enclosed CD.

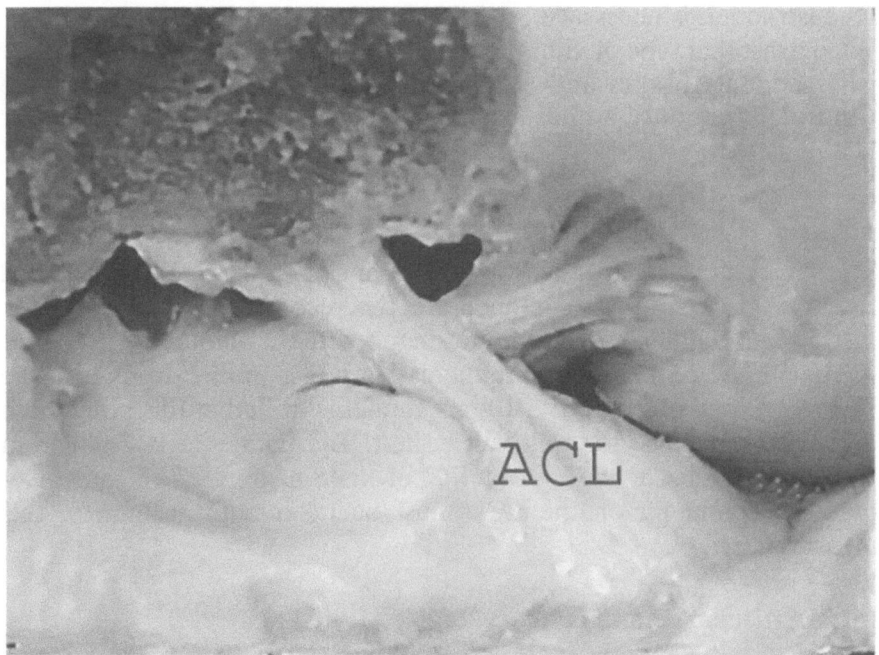

FIGURE 1.2. The ACL is the main restraint to anterior motion of the tibia on the femur.

Biomechanics

Tensile Strength

Noyes has reported the ultimate failure load to be 1750 N. He also noted that the young cadaver specimens were stronger than the older ones.

Viscoelasticity

The speed of the force applied to the ligament affects the type of tear. The slow, twisting type of low-velocity injury experienced by skiers may elongate the ligament it ruptures up to 30%. There may be partial rupture of the anteromedial bundle, leaving the posterolateral bundle intact or vice versa.

If the patient is involved in low-demand activities, this partial remnant may be adequate for stability. We followed 20 recreational athletes diagnosed as having a partial tear. After two years, only one required a reconstruction of the ACL. This one may have been a partial tear or partial healing of a complete tear, but the result is no demonstrable laxity. In high-demand athletes, the bundle may be insufficient to control the pivotal stress and may have to be reconstructed. The conventional wisdom states that if more than 50% of the ligament is still intact, no reconstruction is necessary.

Contrast that type of injury to that of the football or basketball player who suddenly brakes and changes direction. This high-velocity force will usually produce a midsubstance tear, which has little potential for healing.

The Isometric Points

The surgeon must know the isometric points of insertion of the tibia and femur to drill the proper tunnels for the reconstruction of the ACL. Larson and Siddles have computer mapped these points.

The middle of the femoral tunnel is 7 mm in from the drop-off at the 11 or 1 o'clock position. If a 10-mm tunnel is drilled at this point, then a 1- to 2-mm posterior wall will be left. The tibial site is 7 mm from the leading edge of the PCL at 70° of knee flexion. The ligament of Humphrey and fat on the PCL must be taken into account in this measurement.

Intra-Articular Length

The average length of the intra-articular ACL is 31 mm. This is important to know when preparing the length of the semitendinosus and patellar tendon grafts. The total length of the tibial tunnel, the intra-articular length, and the femoral tunnel must be compared to the graft length to avoid mismatch in the endoscopic reconstruction. This calculation avoids protrusion of the graft on the tibial side. The overall length of the graft is 9 to 10cm.

Natural History of ACL Injuries

In his textbook, *Knee Ligaments, Structure, Function, Injury, and Repair*, Dale Daniel describes the fate of the unoperated knee ligament injury. The data come from 500 patients who came to the Kaiser emergency room in San Diego with knee injuries.

Many authors have stated that the ACL injury is career ending for the athlete and that the knee will embark on a course of progressive degeneration. Noyes, however, reported in 1983 on a group of symptomatic patients that he placed on a conservative program of exercise, bracing, and activity modification. From this study came the "rule of thirds." One-third of the patients were able to compensate and return to light sports without symptoms, one-third had to significantly reduce their activities, and one-third required reconstruction. Only 10% of the patients returned to sports without problems.

In Daniel's San Diego study of 279 patients with an isolated ACL injury, 20% underwent acute reconstruction, 18% underwent subsequent reconstruction because of chronic symptoms, and the remainder were treated nonoperatively. This group was followed for at least 5 years. Daniel drew the following conclusions from this study:

- The acute ACL tear is associated with a meniscal tear in 50% of the cases (lateral tears are more frequent than medial tears).
- In the chronic cases, the incidence of tears is 80%. The medial tear is more common in the chronic situation.
- 40% of the tears are repairable.
- Chondral injuries are twice as common (40%) in the chronic cases as compared to the acute cases.
- The patients have minimal pain and no giving way with normal activities of daily living.

The study further concluded that the outcome of the ACL injury is related to the following risk factors:

- *The age of the athlete.* The younger patient did not fare as well as the older patient.
- *The level of sports activity.* The more pivotal sports, such as basketball, volleyball, and soccer, had a higher incidence of inability to par-

ticipate after an ACL injury. This was also related to the level of competition and the number of hours of sports participation.

- *Degree of anteroposterior (a-p) laxity.* Daniel also determined that with more a-p laxity, the functional level of the athlete decreased. He advocated an objective measurement of the laxity with the KT-1000 arthrometer. He determined that more than 3 mm of side-to-side difference was diagnostic of an ACL injury in 98% of the cases. With more than 7 mm of difference and a gross pivot shift examination, he suggested surgical reconstruction.

Mechanisms of Injury

Noncontact Pivot, Internal Rotation/External Rotation

The most common injury mechanism involves no contact with others. The athlete is simply running and abruptly changes direction. The ACL is stressed by the rotation of the tibia, resulting in a tear of the ACL, as illustrated in the video on the CD. The athlete lands in the flexed position, the quadriceps contract, and the tibia is subluxed anteriorly. Then with further flexion, the tibia reduces with a snap. This is the same mechanism that the pivot-shift test mimics. Ireland has reported that the noncontact mechanism is responsible for 80% of ACL tears.

The Quadriceps Active Mechanism

The quadriceps contraction may be of importance in injuring the ACL. Barrett and coworkers have calculated that an eccentric quadriceps contraction can generate up to 6000 N. This far exceeds the strength of the ACL at 1700 N. This force can be observed in basketball in the jump-stop landing. Ireland believes that there is a "position of no return" for ACL injury. The body position is body forward-flexed, hip-abducted, knee that is internally/externally rotated with valgus; the foot is pronated. This position can be reviewed in the video of the badminton player.

However, some additional unrecognized factor must be involved in this mechanism. Many athletes have done that particular move a thousand times without injury. Then, one particular time, the ACL tears. Ireland calls this a "heart attack of the knee." There must be late activation of the hamstrings, because contraction of the hamstrings would normally protect the tibia from subluxing forward.

Barrett and coworkers have reproduced this mechanism of active quadriceps contraction in the laboratory. In the video, the cadaver knee is clamped, the quadriceps mechanism is held with the dry ice clamp, and the force of pulling on the quadriceps subluxes the tibia forward and ruptures the ACL. The next sequence shows the ruptured ACL. The last sequence demonstrates a positive Lachman test on the specimen.

In summary, the body and knee must be in the correct position, the quadriceps must contract strongly enough to sublux the tibia, and the hamstrings fail to protect the anterior subluxation.

Can this be prevented? Perhaps by neuromuscular, proprioceptive training, some injuries may be prevented.

Contact Mechanism

A common mechanism in football or hockey is the blow to the outside of the knee when the knee is flexed and rotated. This initially injures the medial collateral ligament (MCL), and then, with further valgus, the ACL is torn.

Another variation of the contact injury is the internal rotation skiing injury described by Bob Johnson, a doctor from the University of Vermont. In this mechanism, the skier sits back and the ski carves to the inside, producing an internal rotation stress on the knee and a tear of the ACL.

The elements of a potential ACL tear by the contact mechanism are:

- Uphill arm back.
- Skier off balance to the rear.
- Hips below the knees.
- Uphill ski unweighted.
- Weight on the inside edge of downhill ski.
- Upper body generally facing downhill ski.

Johnson has also described another mechanism that occurs when the tail of the ski hits a bump on the snow and the high ski boot levers the tibial forward, thereby producing an anterior drawer force and tearing the ACL.

Hyperflexion or Hyperextension Mechanisms

These less-common mechanisms of injury are often associated with other injuries to ligaments, such as the posterior cruciate ligament.

Gender Issues

During the past decade, the incidence of ACL injury in female athletes has increased more than the rate in male athletes. According to Arendt's study, the injury rates in the National Collegiate Athletic Association

(NCAA) are 2.4 times greater in soccer and 4.1 times greater in basketball for female athletes. The reason is still speculative, but several theories are under investigation. Arendt's statistics show that the noncontact injury mechanism was the main cause of the ACL tear.

In an article by Traina and Bromberg, the authors listed the following as possible causative factors:

Extrinsic
- Muscular strength.
- Body movement.
- Shoe surface interface.
- Level of skill.

Intrinsic
- Joint laxity.
- Limb alignment.
- Notch width and ligament size.

Extrinsic Conditioning

Many authors believe that the novice female athlete is introduced to activities that are beyond her physical conditioning. Tim Hewett has demonstrated that unconditioned females land from a jump with the knee more extended, and, because of the wide pelvis, in a valgus position. This extended valgus position puts them at risk for an ACL injury. If slight external rotation is added on landing, then they are in a position of no return (as described by Ireland). Hewett has advocated not only conditioning programs, but also instruction on proper landing position (i.e., slightly flexed with knees straight ahead). This is one positive step that can be instituted to reduce the incidence of ACL injuries in females.

Muscular Strength

Woitys (in Griffin et al.) has shown that gender differences exist in muscle strength, muscle recruitment order, and hamstring peak torque times. The implication is that women should emphasize hamstring strengthening to protect the ACL.

Body Movement

Arendt and others have documented that most ACL injuries are the result of noncontact mechanisms. The common mechanisms are:

- Planting and cutting: 29%.
- Straight knee landing: 28%.
- Landing with knee hyperextended: 26%.

Hewett has shown that training the female athlete to modify the landing stance to a flexed neutral knee position has reduced the incidence of ACL injuries.

Intrinsic Joint Laxity

There are contradictory studies on the role of ligamentous laxities. Daniel's study with the KT-1000 arthrometer showed no gender differences in the measurable laxity of the ACL. It has been documented that exercise produces laxity of the ACL, but there are no significant differences in gender.

Yu et al. have shown that the ACL has both estrogen and progesterone receptors. The cyclic variation of estrogen may affect the ligament metabolism and make females more prone to injury during the estrogen phase of their cycle. Karangeanes and Vangelos studied the incidence of ACL injury during the cycle of increased estrogen and found no significant difference.

Limb Alignment

Ireland has emphasized limb alignment (the wider pelvis, increased femoral anteversion, and the genu valgum) with decreased muscular support, specifically the hamstrings, as possible causes for the increased ACL injury rates in women

Notch Width

Shelbourne and Klootwyk have documented that women have a smaller notch than men. It has also been reported that athletes who sustain ACL injuries have a narrow notch (Fig. 1.3). It may well be that the narrow notch is only one indication of a small incompetent ligament that is easily torn. Evidence for this is seen after a large notchplasty in which the notch will fill in around the new graft.

Conclusion

At the present time, the best advice to give the female athlete is to be well conditioned and land with a flexed knee.

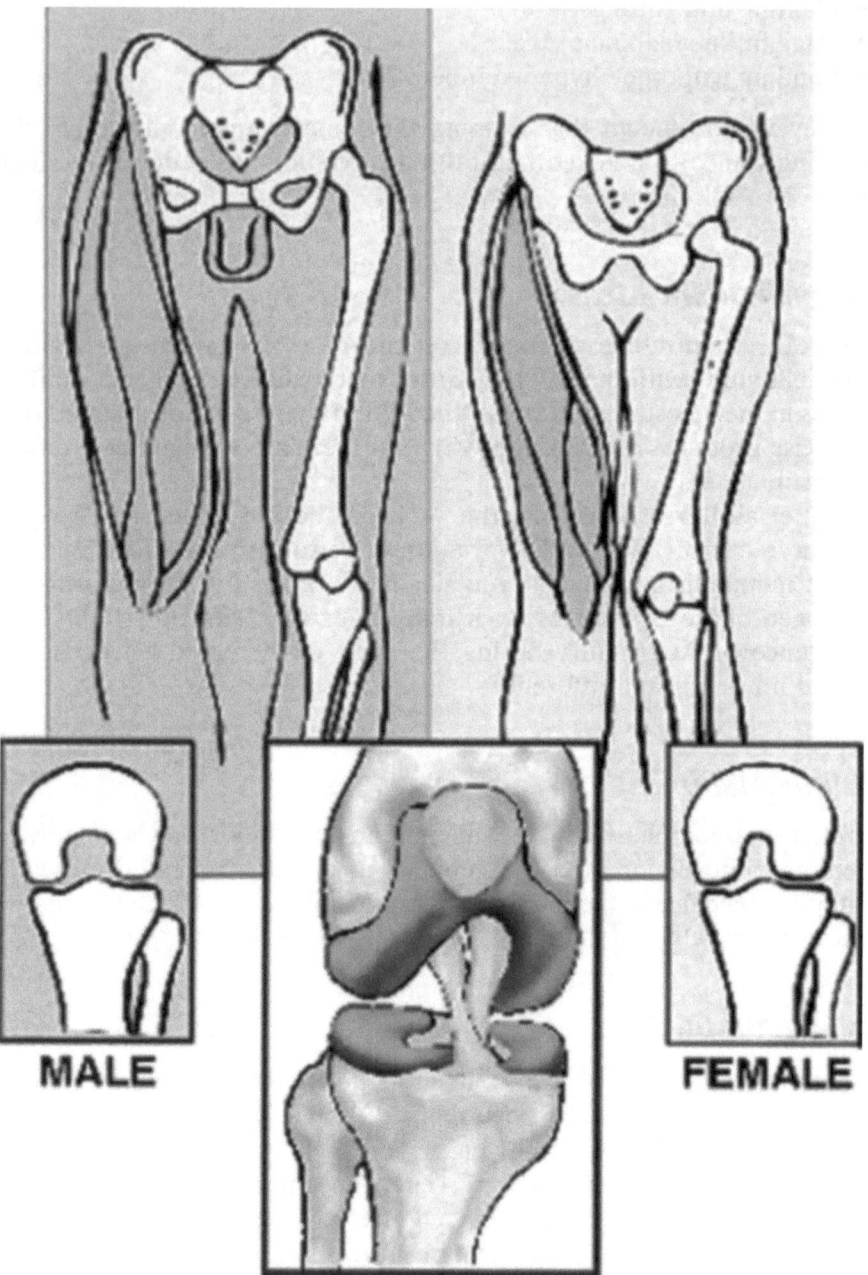

FIGURE 1.3. The anatomic variation of wide pelvis, valgus knees and reduced notch width may increase the risk for ACL injury.

Prevention

Johnson believes that if you are aware of the common mechanism that produces an ACL injury, you can help skiers prevent the injury. He has reviewed thousands of hours of on-hill ski injury video and identified a common mechanism that involves sitting back on the skis and trying to recover as one ski carves inward. The Vermont group has produced a videotape on this mechanism of injury and its prevention. His advice is, do not sit back and then try to recover. Rather, fall to the uphill side. A skier aware of this mechanism may be able to prevent an ACL injury. Johnson has taught the ski patrollers in the area about the mechanism; injury rate has been reduced by 62%.

The phantom foot mechanism and the possible preventive measures have been outlined in a videotape available from Dr. Robert Johnson, University of Vermont, Stafford Hall, Room 426A, Burlington, VT 05405-0084; voice (802) 65-2250; fax (802) 656-4247.

2
Diagnosis of the ACL Injury

History

The athlete describes a twisting injury to his knee, associated with a "popping" sensation in the knee. This is followed by immediate pain and swelling of the knee. He may indicate the feeling of the knee coming apart with the "2-fist sign." Figure 2.1 shows the athlete indicating the "2-fist sign."

The severity of the symptoms vary a great deal, depending on the degree of meniscal, chondral, and capsular injury. The athlete may come in walking, with minimal swelling, or on crutches, unable to bear weight. It depends on the associated injuries.

In rare situations, the injury that tears the anterior cruciate ligament (ACL) may be so trivial that the athlete returns to the game. But the next time he pivots on his knee, much more damage, such as a tear of the meniscus, is the result.

Physical Examination

Lachman Test

The Lachman test is the most definitive and easily performed test for ACL tears (Fig. 2.2). This should be the first test performed, so that the patient can be caught while still relaxed. The knee should be positioned at 20° to 30° of flexion. The upper hand controls the distal thigh, while the lower hand, with the thumb on the tibial tubercle and the fingers feeling to ensure that the hamstrings are relaxed, pulls the tibia forward. The feeling on the normal side is a firm restraint to this anterior motion. The increased excursion on the injured side is noted. When this increased anterior motion is approximately 5 mm and there is a firm endpoint, this should be noted as a 1+ Lachman, with a firm endpoint. This video on the CD demonstrates the Lachman test. In acute injuries,

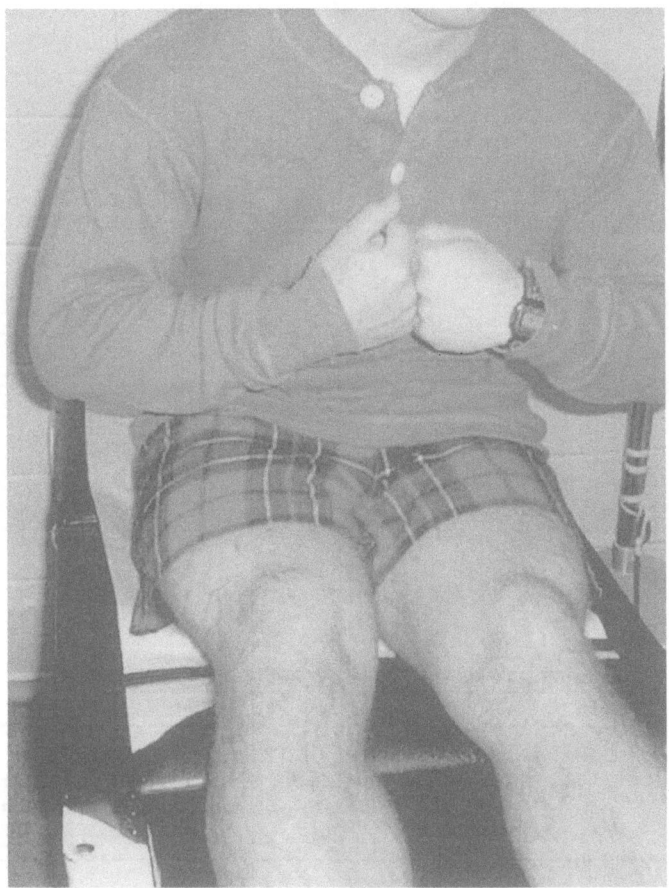

FIGURE 2.1. The "2-fist sign" of ACL instability.

the lower leg should be lowered over the edge of the table to help relax the hamstrings. This position also works well for examiners with small hands or when examining a very large leg. This is called the drop leg test. The ideal knee flexion angle is 30°.

The Lachman test is a subtle test that requires experience to administer confidently. The knee is flexed to 30°, the femur is stabilized, and the tibia is pulled forward. The test is positive when the endpoint is soft. The main feel is the lack of the endpoint to the anterior translation of the tibia. The comparison to the opposite side is important.

The grading should be, negative, 1+ with endpoint, or positive with no endpoint (Table 2.1). It is difficult to differentiate between 2+ and 3+ or to compare between examiners, so these grades have little meaning.

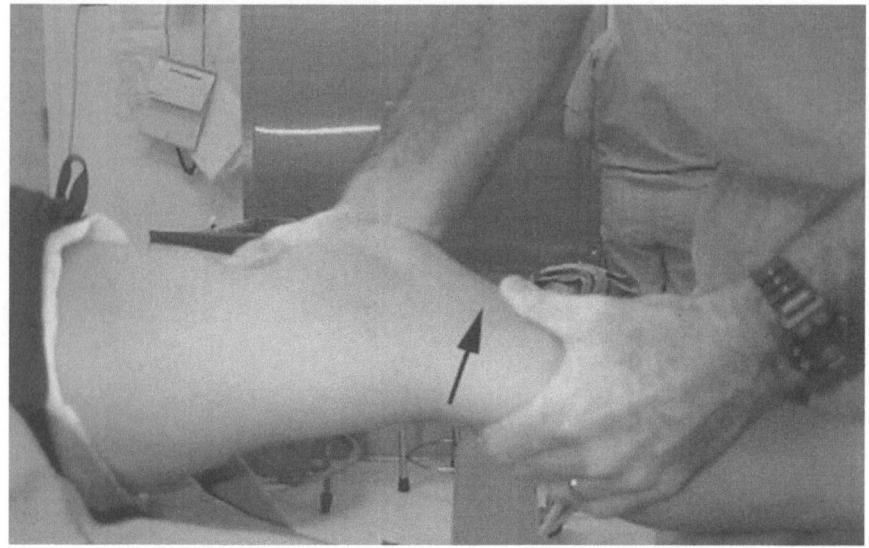

FIGURE 2.2. The Lachman test for ACL laxity.

TABLE 2.1. The Lachman test is graded from 0–3.

Value	Interpretation
0	Negative
1+	0–5 mm of anterior displacement, sometimes with an end point
2+	5–10 mm of anterior displacement, with no end point
3+	10 mm of anterior displacement, with no end point

Pivot-Shift Test

This test is more difficult to perform, but is more consistent in reproducing the athlete's symptoms. Holding the heel in one hand and applying a valgus stress in the other hand, the knee is slowly flexed. The tibia, when in internal rotation, slides anterior when the valgus stress is applied. The tibia, as well as the valgus, subluxes easily if anterior force is applied. After the anterior subluxation of the tibia is noticed, the knee is slowly flexed, and the tibia will reduce with a snap at about 20° to 30° of flexion. This reduction can be augmented with an external rotation of the tibia, as noted in Figure 2.3. This is the "pivot shift." It is the same mechanism that the athlete experiences when his knee "comes apart" with pivoting. The patient will usually indicate that is the sensation experienced when the knee gave out. The pivot-shift test is graded from 0 to 3 (Table 2.2). The video on the CD demonstrates the pivot-shift test.

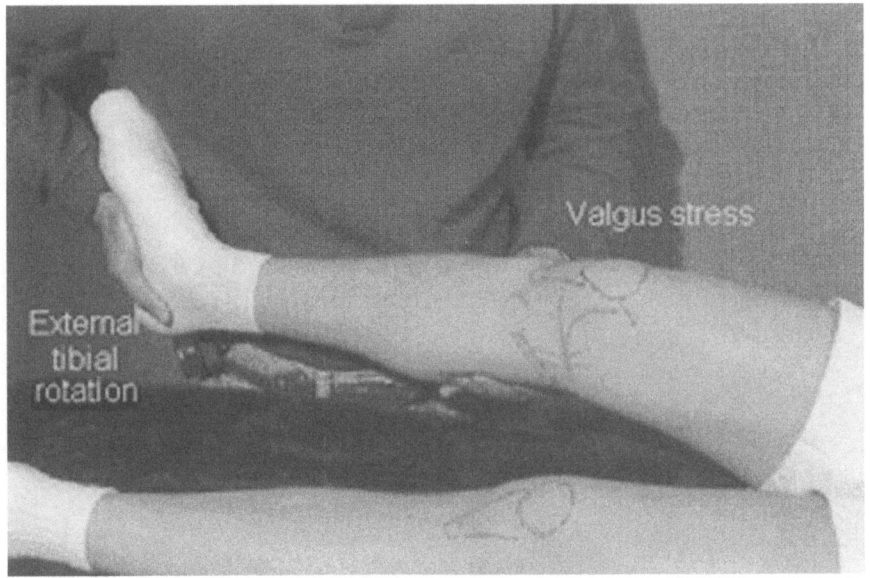

FIGURE 2.3. The pivot-shift test.

TABLE 2.2. The grading of the pivot-shift test.

Value	Interpretation
0	Negative shift
1+	A glide
2+	A pivot shift
3+	A gross pivot shift. where the feeling is that the condyles are dislocated.

Range of Motion

The physician should always examine the knee for loss of extension by holding both heels clear of the table and comparing the extension of the injured knee against the uninjured knee (Fig. 2.4).

The loss of extension is often the result of the ends of the torn ligament impinging anteriorly in the notch. The other common cause of lack of extension is a displaced bucket-handle tear of the meniscus. This may also alert you to a hyperextension and external rotation that indicates an associated posterolateral injury.

Effusion

The tear of the ACL usually produces a hemarthrosis that will appear immediately after the injury. In acute knee injuries, the torn ACL is the

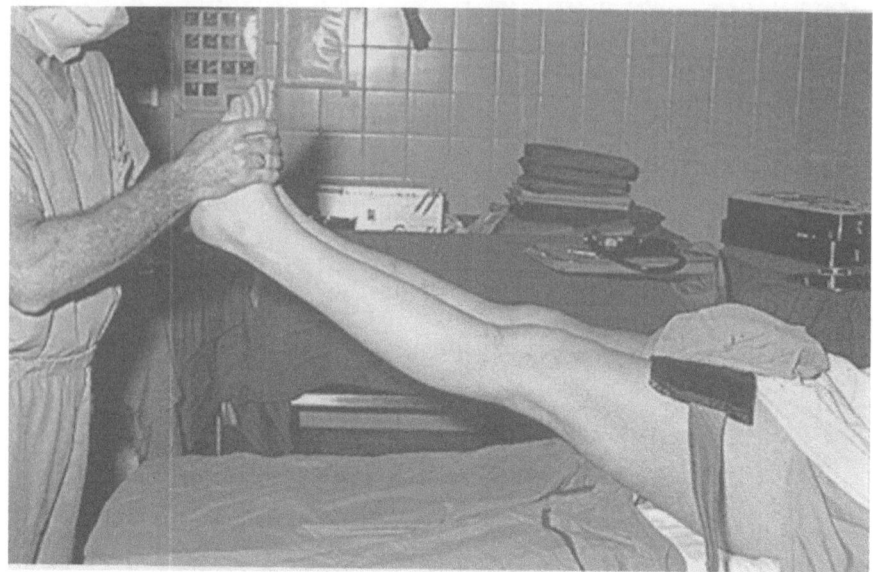

FIGURE 2.4. Both legs are lifted by the heels to examine knee extension.

cause of a bloody effusion in 75% of the cases. This right knee above demonstrates the effusion (Fig. 2.5), noted by the lack of the contour of the patella, which is seen the day after injury.

The acute knee should be aspirated of blood to make the patient

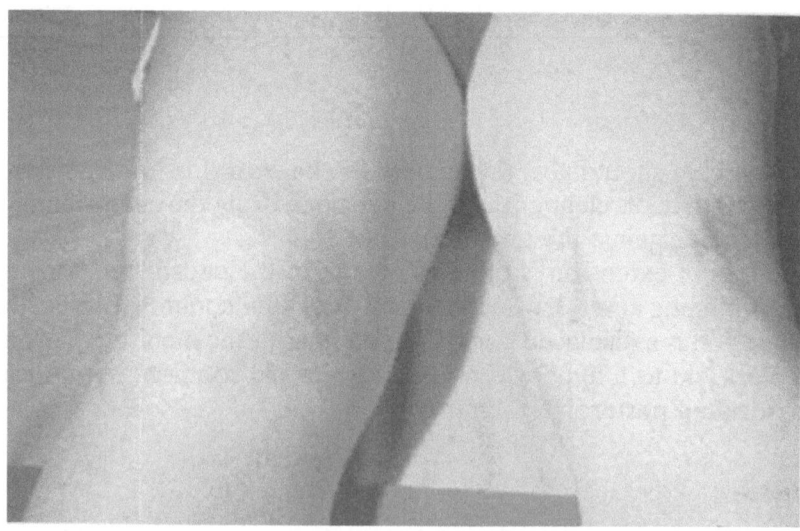

FIGURE 2.5. The right knee demonstrates an effusion.

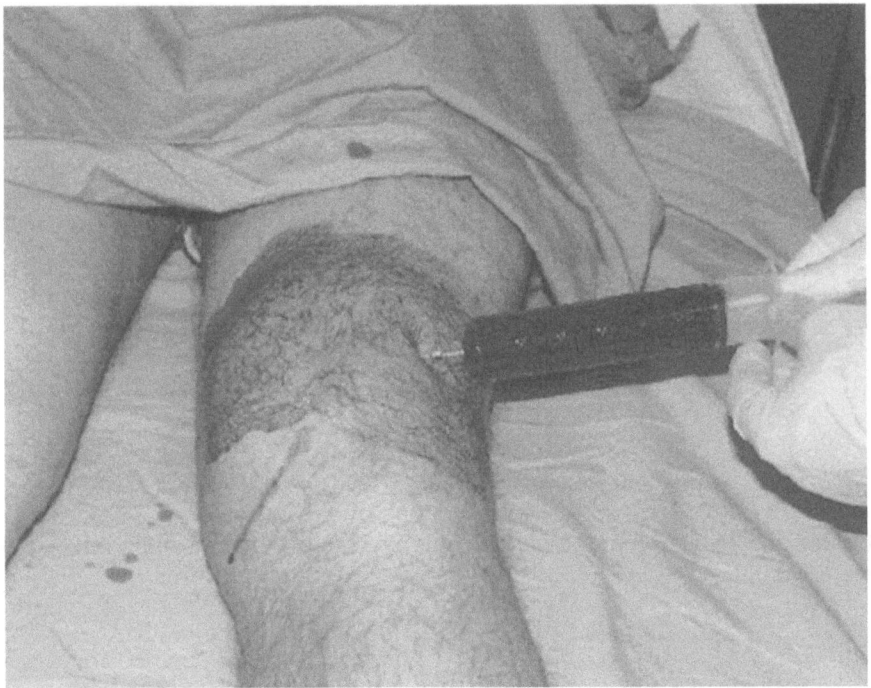

FIGURE 2.6. Aspiration of the hemarthrosis that results from an ACL tear.

more comfortable (Fig. 2.6). If there are visible fat globules on the surface of the blood, this should make you think of an intra-articular fracture. Appropriate imaging studies should be done to detect a tibial plateau fracture.

Joint-Line Tenderness

Both the medial and lateral joint lines should be palpated for tenderness (Fig. 2.7). The meniscal injury usually has joint-line tenderness. In 50% of acute cases, an associated meniscal injury is present. The lateral meniscal tear is more common in the acute situation. In chronic cases, the incidence rises to 80% and is more common on the medial side. In acute cases, it is difficult to do a McMurray test described next because of limited flexion.

McMurray Test

In the chronic situation, the combination of joint-line tenderness, an effusion, and a clunk on the McMurray test confirms a tear of the

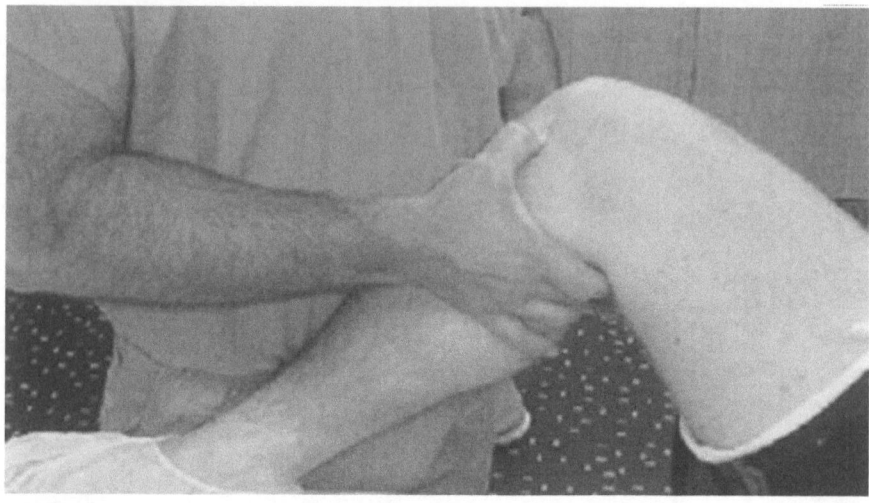

FIGURE 2.7. Palpation of the medial joint line for tenderness compatible with a meniscal injury.

meniscus. The McMurray test is performed by fully flexing the knee and rotating the tibia as the knee is slowly extended (Fig. 2.8). A positive test is painful with full flexion and rotation; a clunk or snap is heard or felt when the knee is extended. The medial tear is elicited initially with the internal rotation followed by the external rotation during extension. The lateral tear is done in the reverse fashion. This rotation of the tibial plateau will catch the posterior horn of the meniscus between the tibia and femoral condyle, producing a clunk and causing pain. The meniscus tugging on the pain-sensitive synovium at its peripheral attachments produces the pain. The test is notoriously inaccurate, and in most situations the pain with full flexion and rotation is sufficient to confirm an injury to the meniscus.

The mechanism of the popping with the McMurray test is demonstrated in the video on the CD. It shows the tibial plateau subluxing forward and trapping the posterior horn of the meniscus between the femur and the tibia. This is associated with a clunk. It also illustrates why the unstable knee has a high incidence of meniscal tears.

Collateral Ligament Assessment

The collateral ligaments are assessed by varus and valgus stress testing at 0° and 30° (Fig. 2.9). The grading is "stable" or "no motion." Grade

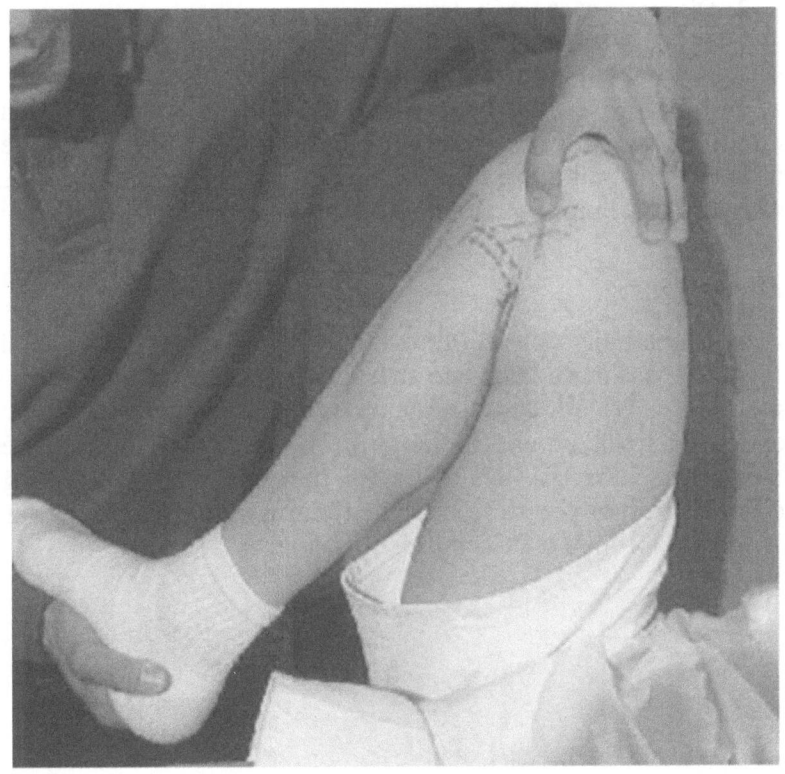

FIGURE 2.8. The McMurray test.

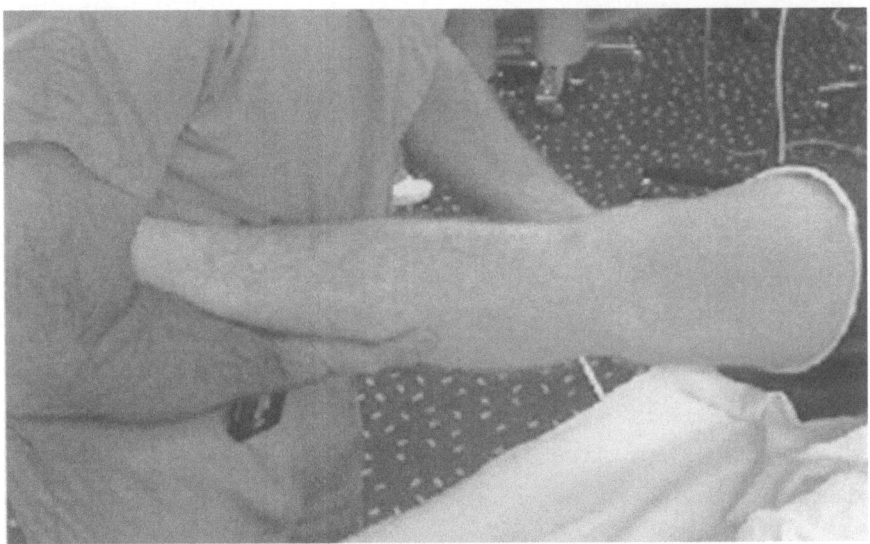

FIGURE 2.9. Valgus stress is applied to the knee to test the medial collateral ligament.

1 has no motion, but is painful on stress. Grade 2 has laxity with an endpoint, and grade 3 is gross laxity at both 0° and 30°. The site of tenderness on the ligament can determine the site of injury (i.e., on the femur or tibia). The examination of the collaterals is important to determine whether the ACL injury is isolated.

Anterior Drawer Test

This test is generally not useful for detecting injury in the acute situation (Fig. 2.10). The drawer becomes positive in the chronic case with capsular laxity. Do not confuse the anterior motion with the knee that is posteriorly subluxed and the anterior motion of pulling the knee to the neutral position. Always check for the tibial step. Examining the knee at 70° reminds you to test for the tibial stepoff. If you routinely do this, you will not miss a PCL injury.

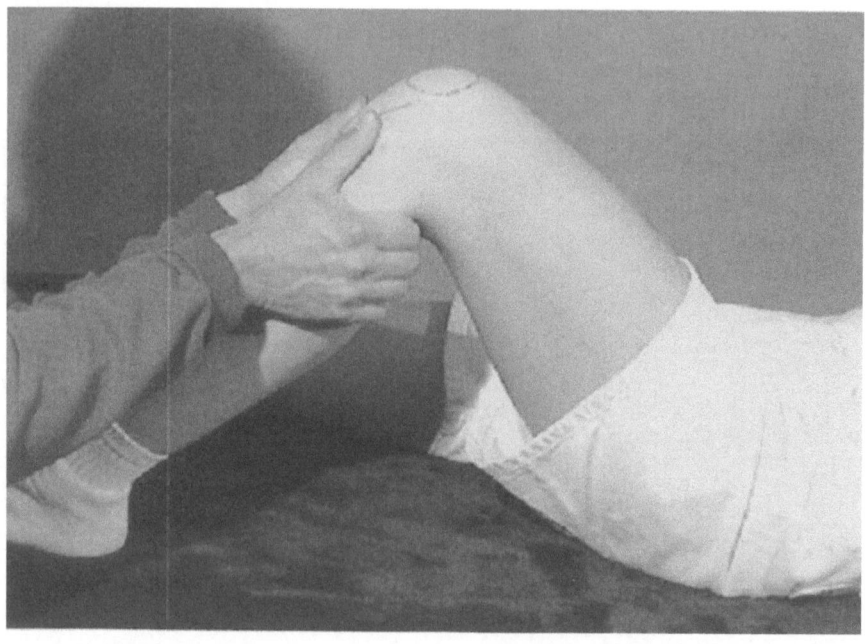

FIGURE 2.10. In the anterior drawer test, the ACL is stressed by pulling the tibia anteriorly at 90° of flexion.

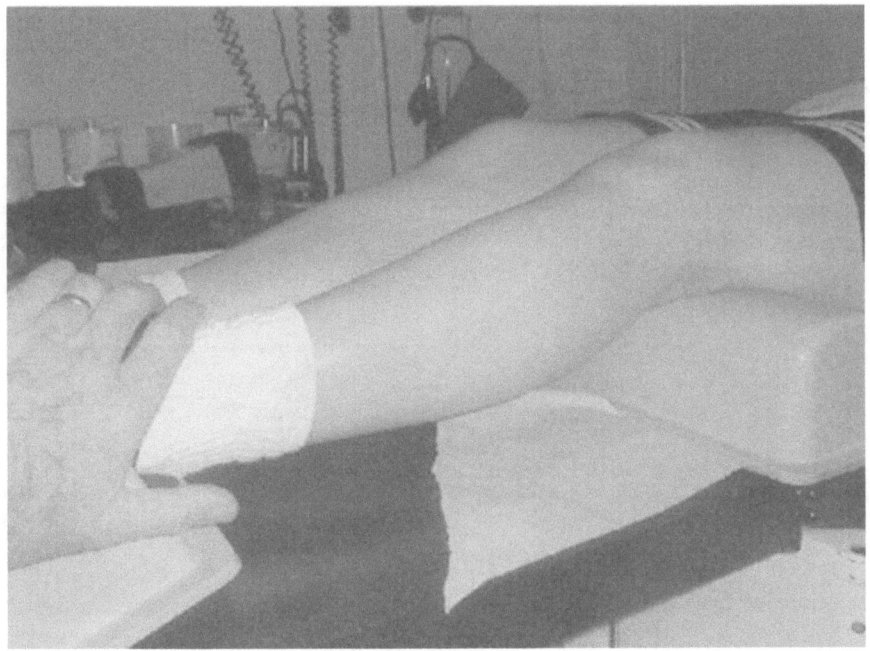

FIGURE 2.11. The active Lachman test.

Quadriceps Active Test

Figure 2.11 shows the left tibia subluxed forward with a quadriceps contraction. This is indicative of an ACL-deficient knee. When the quadriceps is contracted against resistance with the knee flexed at 30° and without weight bearing, there is an anterior displacement of the tibia (this is an open kinetic chain exercise). Figure 2.11 shows the tibia subluxed anteriorly. This nonweight-bearing exercise is called open kinetic chain exercise.

Open kinetic chain exercise is also seen with the patient on the quadriceps machine in a fitness room. The athlete sits on the leg extension machine and extends the knee. The quadriceps pulls the tibia forward if there is no ACL or causes significant strain on the ACL graft. In the early rehabilitation phase, this exercise must be avoided to prevent strain on the recently implanted graft.

Associated Ligament Injuries

It is always important to perform a posterior drawer test (Fig. 2.12). If this is done routinely, you will not miss a posterior cruciate ligament

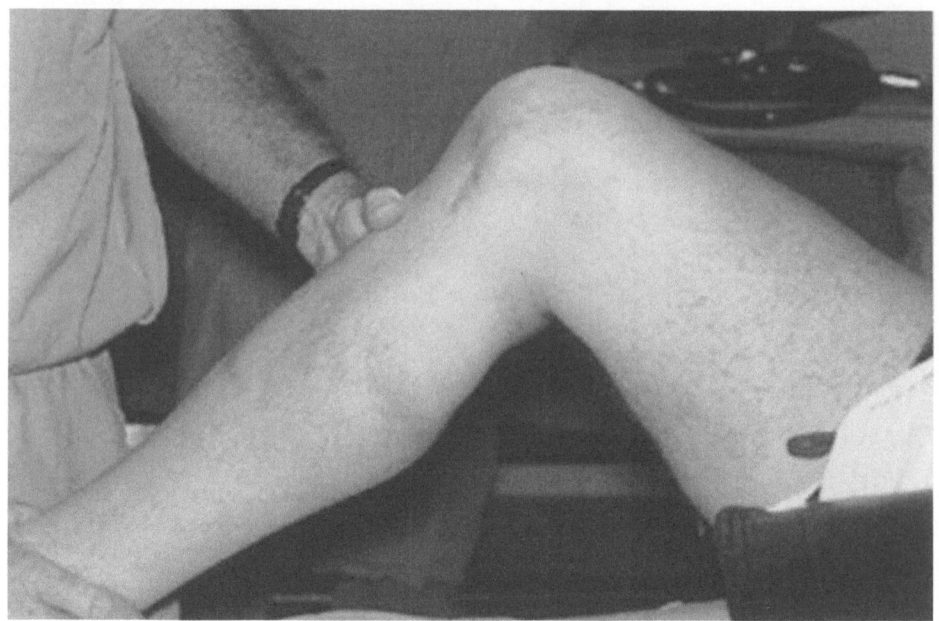

FIGURE 2.12. The posterior drawer test for PCL laxity.

injury. The video on the CD demonstrates the posterior drawer test. The external rotation of the tibia must be measured at both 90° and 30° to rule out associated injury to the posterolateral corner.

Imaging

Plain Radiographs

The screening examination should be a simple anteroposterior and lateral radiograph of the knee. This will reveal open growth plates, ACL bony avulsions, significant osteochondral fractures, tibial plateau fractures, or epiphyseal fractures.

Tomograms

If the radiograph is negative, but considerable bony tenderness exists, then tomograms should be done to rule out plateau fractures.

Computed Tomography Scan

The 3-D scan can help plan treatment for associated tibial plateau fractures.

Bone Scan

If the pain persists, this scan may confirm occult bony injury.

Magnetic Resonance Imaging

In a few situations, magnetic resonance imaging (MRI) will change your management of an injury. The diagnosis of the ACL tear should be made clinically. If the loss of extension persists, the MRI can be performed to determine whether this is a bucket-handle tear or an impingement of the ACL bundle, a cyclops lesion. The meniscus tear should be repaired early and, in some situations, the ACL reconstruction should be delayed until a good range of motion has been achieved after the meniscus repair. In the cyclops lesion, both the debridement of the ligament ends and the ACL reconstruction can be done simultaneously as described by Pinczewski. Remember that a good physical examination by an experienced physician is more reliable than an MRI.

Examination Under Anesthesia and Arthroscopy

The arthroscope has been the key to unlocking the diagnosis of knee pathology (Fig. 2.13). The arthroscope has improved the diagnosis of knee injuries, but the scope examination is only one aspect of the puzzle. One of the mistakes residents make is to go ahead with the arthroscopy before performing a clinical examination of the knee. The examination under anesthesia (EUA) is a valuable adjunct to the diagnostic work-up. At this time, the grading of the laxity may be documented. It is often difficult to examine the very large knee of a football player with multiple ligament injuries in the training room. The EUA may be the only means of making the diagnosis.

Arthroscopy of the acute knee presents no more technical problems than with the elective case. The hemarthrosis must first be flushed out. The synovium and ligamentum mucosum around the ACL must frequently be removed to fully assess the degree of ligament injury. The hook is used to probe the two bundles, and to assess tension.

The video on the CD shows how the diagnostic arthroscopy must be performed in a similar fashion each time, so that the knee will be completely examined and no region forgotten. This must be done before any surgical procedures are started. The video shows the inside view of the "W" arthroscopy. The "W" procedure enables the physician to view the patellofemoral joint, the medial gutter, the medial compartment with the medial meniscus, and then to go over the top of the

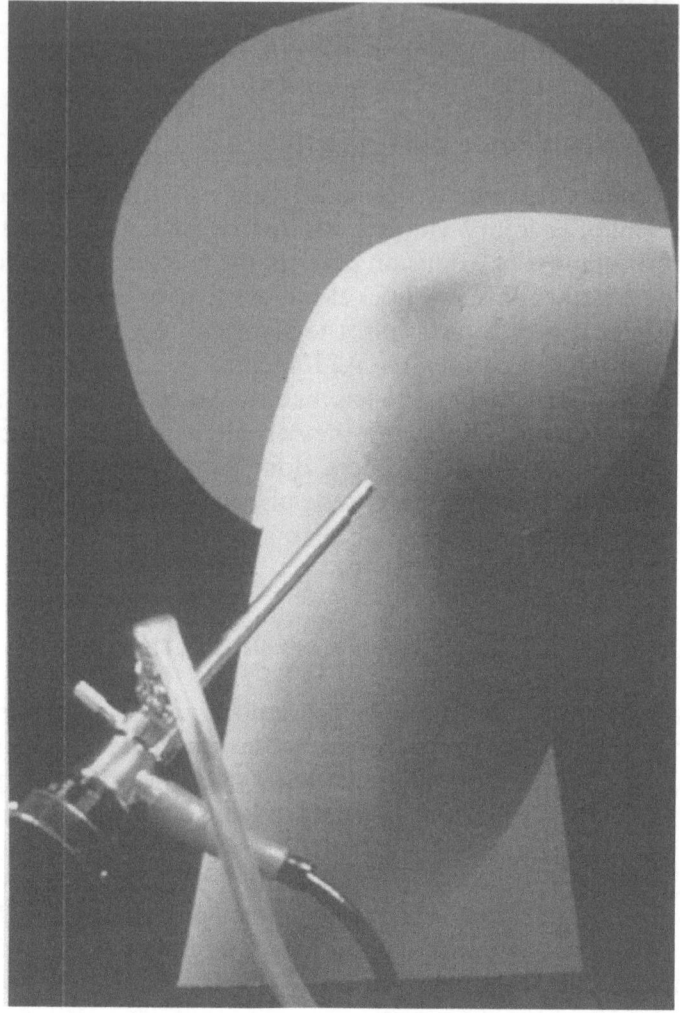

FIGURE 2.13. The arthroscope is the key to unlocking the secrets of the knee.

ligamentum mucosum to view the ACL and finally the lateral compart-ment with the lateral meniscus.

The video shows the arthroscopic view of the torn ACL. The menis-cus and articular surface should be completely examined. The capsular injury may be seen by inspecting the gutters, and examining over and under the meniscus. If there is significant capsular tearing, then gravity pressure only, rather than a pump, should be used. The ACL tear has produced a stump at the front of the knee that prevents full extension. This mimics a locked knee.

This ACL tear is only partial or interstitial. The fat pad in front of the ligament has to be removed to visualize the ligament, and the ligament must be probed to assess its status. This ligament tear may have been produced by the narrow stenotic notch.

The diagnostic examination of the knee must be complete to detect any meniscal injuries. In the acute knee, the incidence of meniscal tear is approximately 50%. In the chronic ACL-deficient knee, the incidence of meniscal tears may be as high as 75%.

The video demonstrates the chronic ACL tear. The residual ligament is probed with a hook, and it can be appreciated that it is not attached to the femoral condyle.

3
Partial Tears of the ACL

One of the dilemmas facing the sports physician is treatment of the partial tear of the anterior cruciate ligament. The definition of a partial tear is a history of injury to the anterior cruciate ligament, a positive Lachman test with a firm end point, a negative pivot-shift test, KT-1000 side-to-side difference of <5 mm, and arthroscopic evidence of injury to the anterior cruciate ligament.

The natural history of the partial tear is controversial. Reports suggest that both conservative and operative treatment offer good results. Noyes and his colleagues had a 50% incidence of instability in high-demand sports participation athletes who had an anterior cruciate ligament tear of more than 50%. They also had a 75% incidence of reinjury. This suggests that patients in high-demand sports require reconstruction. Freunsgaard and Johannsen had good results with conservative treatment in patients who avoided high-demand athletics, and Buckley and colleagues reported that the degree of anterior cruciate tear did not correlate with outcome. Only half of their patients were able to resume their previous level of sports activity.

Physical Examination

Lachman Test

The Lachman test is positive, but there is a firm end point (See Fig. 2.2). This anterior excursion is greater than the opposite side, but less than 5 mm of the side-to-side difference measured on the KT-1000 arthrometer.

Pivot-Shift Test

The pivot-shift test must be negative or only a slight glide to produce a diagnosis of a partial tear (See Fig. 2.3). If the test is positive, the knee is clinically unstable and should be regarded as anterior cruciate deficient. The pivot shift is the most important assessment of the partial tear.

The KT-1000 Arthrometer

The KT-1000 arthrometer will normally show a side-to-side difference of less than 5 mm (Fig. 3.1). The slope of the curves that are pulled with the KT-2000 demonstrate the difference. Force of 15, 20, and 30 pounds is applied to the vertical axis of the knee; the horizontal axis shows millimeters of displacement. The curve on the left shows the normal anterior cruciate ligament. The middle curve shows that there is initially more displacement, but then a firm restraint to anterior translation. This corresponds to the firm end point to the Lachman test. The third curve on the right is the anterior cruciate deficient knee with complete rupture. The stronger the pull, the more anterior displacement.

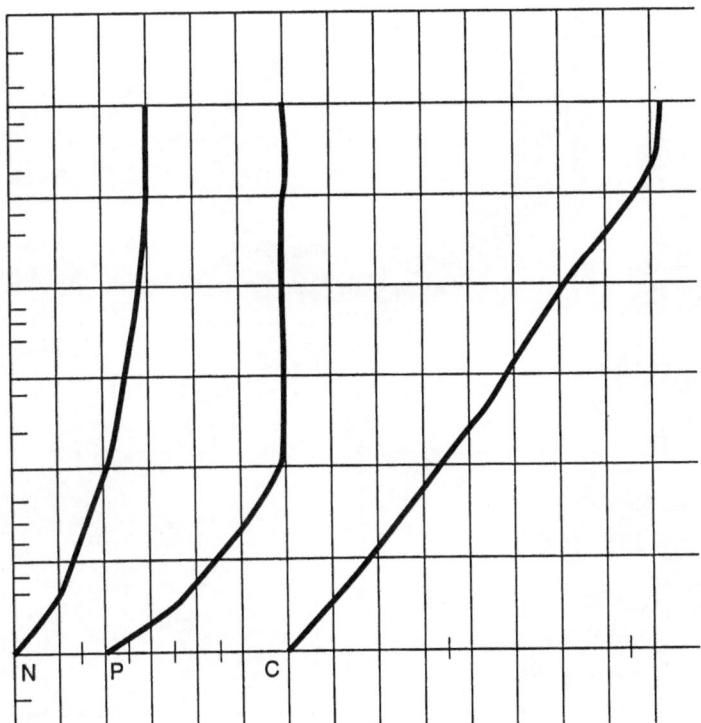

FIGURE 3.1. The force displacement curve of the partial ACL tear.

Magnetic Resonance Imaging

It is difficult to estimate the degree of ACL injury with the MRI, as the laxity of the ligament cannot be accurately assessed. Therefore, it is not a useful tool for diagnosing partial tears of the anterior cruciate ligament. Figure 3.2 shows a small band where the anterior cruciate ligament should be. It is difficult to estimate how much of the ligament is still present.

Arthroscopic Assessment

Arthroscopic assessment of the anterior cruciate ligament tear is difficult for two reasons. First, it is hard to see the ligament without removing the synovium and fat pad. Second, it is only an estimate of the degree of tearing of the ligament. It seems to be best to try to estimate

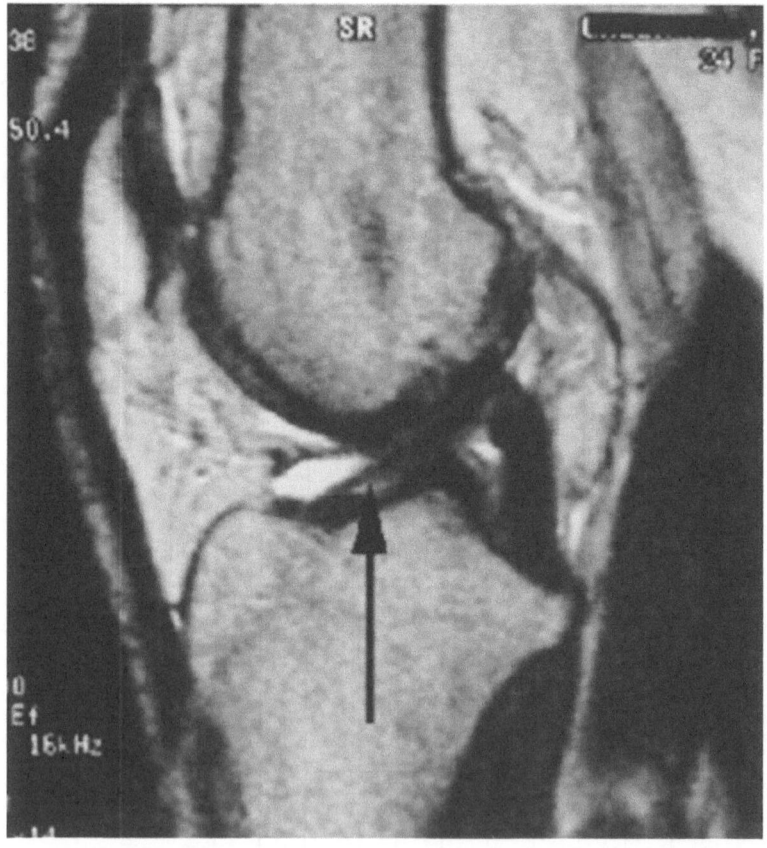

FIGURE 3.2. The MRI imaging of the ACL tear.

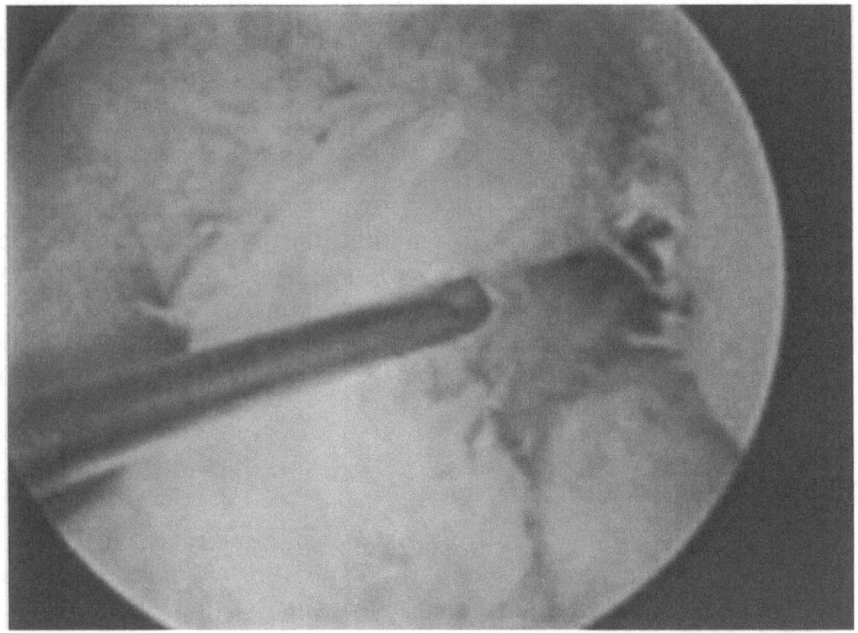

FIGURE 3.3. The laxity of the ACL is demonstrated with a probe.

whether the tear is less than or greater than 50%. A hook probe must be used to examine the ligament proximally to see where the ligament is attached—to the side wall, the roof, or the posterior cruciate ligament. The best position is the side wall at the normal site of the anterior cruciate ligament. The most common situation is to see the ligament attached to the posterior cruciate ligament.

Figure 3.3 shows the appearance of the ligament proximally. It has attenuated to a small band attached to the side wall. This may give a 1+ Lachman test and a negative pivot-shift test, but would not stand up to vigorous pivoting activities. Figure 3.3 also shows the use of the probe to examine the ligament proximally. This example is lax, but is less than 50% tear. This amount of ligament laxity should allow a return to sports without a reconstruction.

Treatment Options

Partial Tears

The treatment options for a patient with partial ACL tear are to give up or modify his or her sports activities. The patient who can modify his sports activities and avoid pivotal sports will do well with a partial anterior cruciate ligament injury. This is the only parameter that the individual has control over, and that point should be emphasized when counseling athletes.

Brace and Arthroscopy

The use of a brace combined with modification of activity can be successful. Sometimes a meniscal injury will still cause a giving way sensation. The best long-term outcome for the young patient is to have a meniscal repair. The dilemma is whether to reconstruct the ACL. The results of a meniscal repair are much better when the knee has been reconstructed and is stable.

ACL Reconstruction

If there is a positive pivot-shift test or a small bundle attached to the femur, and the athlete wants to be active in pivoting sports, anterior cruciate ligament reconstruction should be considered.

Indications for ACL Reconstruction

The patient who is a candidate for reconstruction of the ACL is the competitive, pivoting athlete who is involved in sports such as soccer, rugby, and basketball. In addition, the patient should have clinical symptoms of instability, with a history of giving way, a positive Lachman, and pivot-shift test with more than 5 mm side-to-side difference on the KT-1000 arthrometer.

4
Treatment Options for ACL Injuries

The treatment of the anterior cruciate injury must be individualized to the patient. Not all tears of the ACL need operative repair. The treatment options for the elite athlete, who needs reconstruction, as well as the inactive patient, who needs no reconstruction, are fairly limited. It is the recreationally active individual whose ACL injury requires counseling for the best treatment plan. There are a number of factors to consider in this decision, including, as Shelbourne has emphasized, age, chronicity, activity level, and associated injury to the meniscus and articular surface.

Patient Factors

The treatment of the ACL injury should be determined by the following factors.

Age of the Patient

The older patient may be more likely to modify his lifestyle and accept a conservative treatment program, while the younger patient, who is involved in competitive sports, wants to return as quickly as possible to high-level sports without the use of a brace.

Activity Level and Intensity

The competitive football or soccer player will likely require a reconstruction to continue playing at the same level. Noyes has shown that only 10% of nonoperatively treated athletes go back to the same level of sport activities.

Degree of Instability

In the Kaiser study, the outcome was related to degree of instability. If the KT-1000 arthrometer side-to-side difference was greater than 7 mm, the chance of a better outcome was with surgical reconstruction.

Size of Athlete

The forces that a 300 lb lineman exerts on his knee with pivoting are much more that the 150 lb tennis player. In the case of the former, surgical reconstruction should be considered.

Treatment Choices

There are 3 treatment choices for the ACL tear.

Give Up or Modify Sport Activities

It is important to emphasize that the ACL is asymptomatic with most activities of daily living. If the patient is not involved in sports then he will usually have no giving way episodes, and no surgical treatment is necessary. Giving way in the sedentary patient is more likely the result of meniscal pathology. The meniscus may be treated by arthroscopy, and the patient can continue with the nonoperative treatment program. The patient should be counseled to switch into knee friendly sports, such as cycling and swimming.

Brace and Arthroscopic Meniscectomy

If the patient is recreationally active, a functional brace will often be sufficient to stabilize the knee for low-demand sports, such as doubles tennis. However if he has giving way in the brace, a meniscal tear may be present. Approximately 50% of ACL tears have an associated meniscal tear. The younger athlete should have a meniscal repair and reconstruction for the ACL. The long-term results of meniscal repair are better with a stable knee, and the meniscal repair without reconstruction is not an option. The older patient should have a meniscectomy and use a brace for sports. If the patient still gives way in the brace, then consideration should be given to a reconstruction.

Anterior Cruciate Ligament Reconstruction

Most young competitive, pivoting athletes should have an ACL reconstruction to stabilize their knees. This will allow them to continue to participate in sports and, hopefully, prevent late degenerative changes. Shelbourne has recently reported that if the meniscus and articular cartilage is normal at the index operation, the X-ray evaluation will be normal at 10 years in 97% of the patients. This means that the athlete who has an early ACL reconstruction will be able to continue to be active without the risk of degenerative osteoarthritic changes in his knee. The patient who continues in sports with recurrent giving way, as a result of ACL laxity, will have a degenerative knee in 10 to 12 years.

Summary

The most important outcome factors are the patient's age, the activity level, and the degree of instability. The activity level is the only one of these factors that the patient can control. Thus for a nonoperative approach to be successful, the patient's activity level must be modified. The other treatment options, such as brace and meniscal repair, will only be successful if activity is diminished. Ninety percent of the patients who undergo ACL reconstruction will be able to return to full athletic participation.

Plea for Conservative Treatment

Conventional wisdom states that the ACL does not heal. However, in some instances, especially with downhill skiing injuries, it can. There is little argument that the young competitive, pivoting soccer player with a positive pivot shift and a 7-mm side-to-side difference on the KT arthrometer needs a reconstruction, but consider another example.

Case 1

KB, who is a 31-year-old interior designer and an advanced recreational skier, injured her knee downhill skiing. She had an external rotation, valgus injury with an audible pop in her knee. The bindings did not release. She was assessed at the ski hill and diagnosed with an ACL tear. Two weeks later, an examination at the clinic revealed an effusion, joint-line tenderness, positive Lachman, and a positive pivot-shift test. She was advised to have a reconstruction and started therapy to improve the range of motion and reduce the effusion. At six weeks after injury, she had a positive Lachman (no end point), positive pivot shift, and a KT manual maximum side-to-side difference of 6 mm. She was advised to proceed with a reconstruction.

At three months postinjury, she had a positive Lachman with a firm end point, a pivot glide, and a KT manual maximum side-to-side dif-

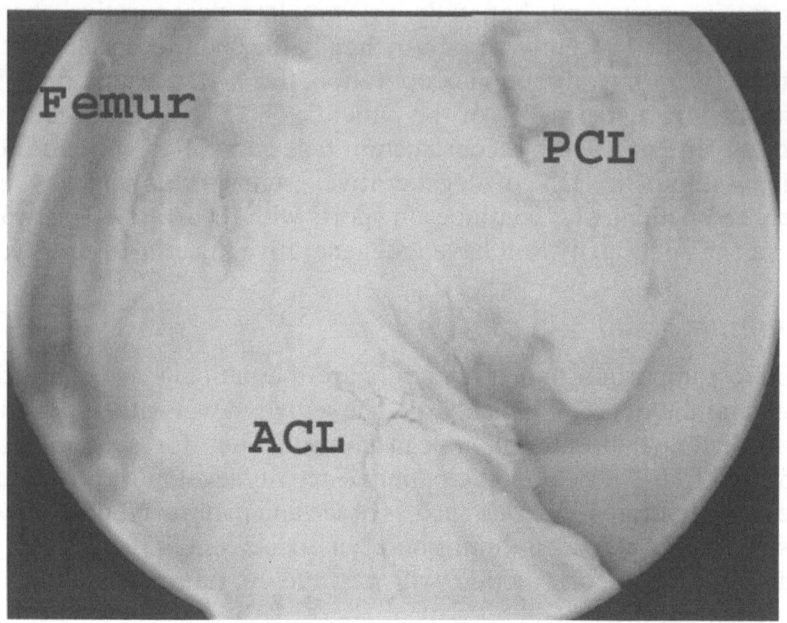

FIGURE 4.1. The arthroscopic appearance of a healed ACL.

ference of 2mm. The arthroscopic examination demonstrated normal
menisci, normal articular cartilage, and an ACL healed to the femoral
condyle. The appearance of the well-healed ACL is shown in Figure 4.1.

We have usually divided the degree of injury to the ACL as more than
or less than 50%. In reality, this means a normal appearing bulk of
ligament present as opposed to this thin strand of ligament. Figure 4.2
shows the arthroscopic appearance of a small incompetent band of ACL
left after partial healing of the ACL tear. No physician would have a
problem proceeding with a reconstruction in this situation.

Conclusion

On the basis of the clinical examination alone, a physician could probably recommend conservative treatment of this injury. However, what
the physician cannot assess is how much of the ligament is present. If
the patient described above had only the small strand shown in Figure
4.2, would it be wise to allow her to go back to aggressive skiing, to pos-
sibly reinjure her knee and tear her meniscus?

Yet, a number of skiing patients who have torn the ACL have been
documented with clinical examinations and with KT arthrometer read-
ings that eventually heal and do not require surgery. In the past, surgery

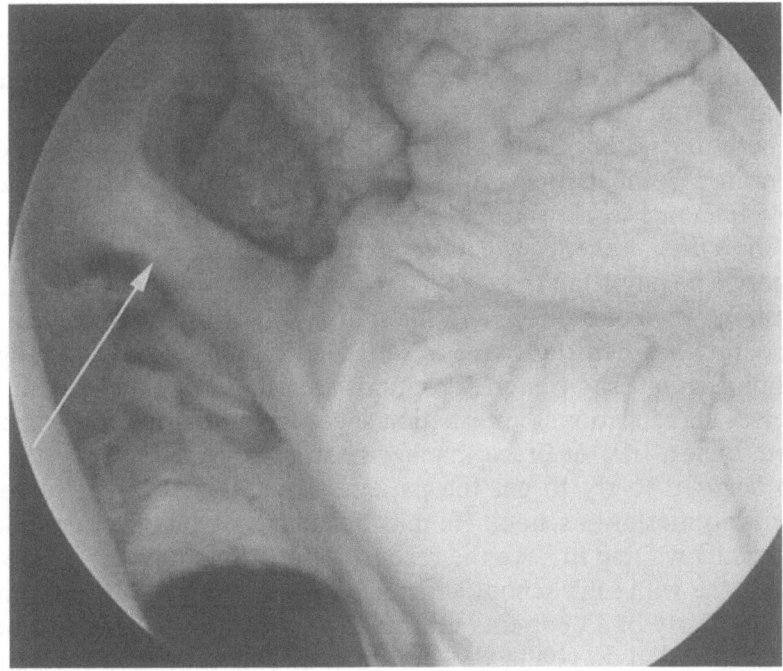

FIGURE 4.2. The arthroscopic appearance of a partial healing of an ACL tear.

would have taken place within the first few weeks of the injury, and there would have been no opportunity to see this natural evolution of the healing process.

Timing of Surgical Intervention

The timing of surgical treatment is controversial. Shelbourne has shown that reconstruction done acutely results in more stiffness and greater loss of range of motion. To avoid this, reconstruction should be delayed until a full range of motion is achieved. In the Sports Medicine Clinic, after the diagnosis is made, most patients go to physiotherapy to regain range of motion and to reduce the swelling. No one is reconstructed without full knee extension. If full extension is not gained in physiotherapy, then the torn ACL bundle or a bucket-handle tear of the meniscus must be treated first. Arthroscopy should be performed to repair the meniscus or excise the cyclops lesion of the ACL before the reconstruction. After the meniscal tear is repaired or excised, physiotherapy is resumed to regain knee extension before the reconstruction. Pinczweski has reported that the cyclops lesion of the ACL may be removed and the ACL reconstruction done at the same time without risk of limited motion postoperatively, but Shelbourne recommends that repair of the bucket-handle meniscus tear and the ACL reconstruction should be staged.

There are no hard and fast rules, such as wait three weeks before operating. Some patients will have good range of motion and no swelling in one week, and they need only to work on the bike preoperatively. Other patients will take six or eight weeks to be ready for surgery. The physician should read the tissues. This means to look at the effusion, range of motion, and the induration of the capsule. The time to operate is when the tissue is soft and compliant, and the range of motion is good. The treatment options are outlined to the patient, who receives an educational information sheet on the options. If he is undecided, then a trial of brace management is suggested. The brace may also be used to try to get the patient through the current season of sport or semester of school. He may be able to participate at a reduced level while waiting to have the reconstruction. Shelton has reported his experience with high school athletes who tear their ACLs early in the season. Thirty of 43 patients returned to play in 6 weeks with a brace, but only 12 had no giving way episodes. Twenty-nine of these patients eventually underwent ACL reconstruction. The downside of this experience is that some of these patients were unable to undergo meniscal repair because of further injury of the meniscus. It is also important to reexamine and remeasure the KT-1000, as some of these patients will partially heal to a 1+ Lachman. This partial healing may be adequate stability for the recreational athlete.

Controversial Treatment Decisions

Other factors that influence the decision to treat are associated lesions, such as chondral fractures, meniscal tears, and other ligament tears, but the real controversies center on the age of the patient, the associated injury to the medial collateral ligament, and the patient with medial compartment osteoarthritis.

Older Athlete

Age is, in many ways, the least important factor. The most important is the activity level of the individual, and the next is the degree of instability, or degree of a-p translation. Nowadays, surgical treatment should not be reserved only for the "young, competitive, pivotal" athlete. With very active "mature" athletes, forty years of age is not a contraindication for surgery. Patient selection may be expanded according to activity level. The younger and more pivotal athlete, who wants to return to sport sooner may be a candidate for the patellar tendon graft. Shelbourne has reported on return to sports at four months with a contralateral patellar tendon graft harvest.

Older, more recreational athletes usually have a semitendinosus autograft graft or an allograft patellar tendon. There have been several authors, including Brandsson, who have reported positive results of ACL reconstruction in patients more than 40 years of age. Remember that the patellar tendon graft is for the surgeon, and the semitendinosus graft is for the patient.

Immature Athlete

Anterior cruciate ligament injuries in skeletally immature adolescents are being diagnosed with increasing frequency. Nonoperative management of midsubstance ACL injuries in adolescent athletes frequently results in a high incidence of giving-way episodes, recurrent meniscal tears, and early onset of osteoarthritis. In the past, the protocol has been to recommend conservative treatment until the growth plates have closed. Shelbourne has reported that an intra-articular ACL reconstruction (using the central 10-mm patellar tendon graft) in young athletes approaching skeletal maturity provides predictable excellent knee stability, and the athletes are able to return to competitive sports with a decreased risk of recurrent meniscal and/or chondral injury. The patients can be divided into prepubescent and postpubescent. The latter are treated in the usual fashion; the former are a treatment dilemma. Because very young athletes (i.e., those less than 12 years of age) do not modify or restrict their activities, they are usually not good candidates for this initial conservative treatment. The concern about ACL reconstruction in the athlete with open growth plates is that there will be premature fusion of the plate, growth arrest, and potential for angular deformities. DeLee and others have recommended procedures that avoid crossing the growth plates with tunnels. This type of procedure and other extra-articular operations, however, achieve less than satisfactory stability. Stadelmaier, Arnoczsky, and others have shown in the laboratory that a tunnel drilled centrally across the growth plate and filled with a tendon does not cause growth arrest of the epiphyseal plate. Based on this basic research, several clinicians have reported on a series of young patients with small central tunnels placed through both the femur and tibia and the semitendinosus graft. The tunnels are drilled centrally through the epiphysis and fixed with a button on the periosteal surface. There are no reported growth deformities with this technique.

The two options to consider with the nine-year-old patient who tears his ACL is restriction of activity and the use of a brace until skeletal maturity. Then consider an intra-articular reconstruction versus an early reconstruction using the semitendinosus graft and button fixation.

ACL/MCL Injuries

The management of the combined ACL/MCL injury is controversial. This is a common injury seen among skiers who catch an inside edge and externally rotate the knee. Shelbourne has advocated initial conservative treatment of the MCL, followed by ACL reconstruction as indicated. Our current protocol at the Sports Medicine Clinic is to treat the MCL with an extension splint, or brace, until it is stable. Then the patient works to regain range of motion and strength, after which reconstruction of the ACL, if necessary, can be performed. After the medial collateral ligament heals, the degree of partial healing of the ACL is usually sufficiently stable for recreational activities. This patient will often not require surgical reconstruction.

The dilemma occurs when there is residual laxity of both the MCL and the ACL. In this situation, the patient will have significant symptoms with pivotal activity. The treatment is a custom-made functional brace with double upright support. If there are still instability symptoms, reconstruction of the ACL must be performed. The MCL may be treated in a variety of ways. The course of the ligament may be picked with an awl to produce bleeding and microfracture of the ligament attachment. This produces scarring and shortening of the MCL. This is an option for a mild degree of laxity. The next level of treatment is to plicate the ligament with sutures. The attachment site of the MCL on the femur may be removed with an osteotomy and countersunk into the femur about 1 cm to shorten the ligament. The bone plug is held with a staple. The posterior capsule is plicated to this post of retensioned ligament. In severe cases of laxity, the ligament is shortened and reinforced with an autograft or allograft of semitendinosus. A brace must be used in the postoperative protocol to protect this MCL reconstruction for a prolonged period.

Osteoarthritis and the ACL Deficient Knee

There are three clinical presentations with combined ACL laxity and medial compartment osteoarthritis. The first is the patient with primarily ACL laxity symptoms; that is, recurrent giving way and mild activity related pain. This is best treated with an ACL reconstruction alone. The second is the patient with more severe osteoarthritis and ACL laxity. The symptoms are pain and giving way associated with a varus knee and medial compartment narrowing on the standing X-rays. This patient should be managed with a combined ACL reconstruction and tibial osteotomy done at the same sitting. It is acceptable to stage the osteotomy as the initial procedure, followed by the ligament reconstruction six months later. The third scenario is the patient with advanced medial compartment osteoarthritis and residual ACL laxity. The injury usually is long standing; the knee is in varus, but lacks extension. The patient at this point has pain, but not giving way. The best treatment is a tibial osteotomy. The closing wedge osteotomy of Coventry has been the standard, but the opening wedge osteotomy is becoming popular.

Nonoperative Management Protocol

The nonoperative treatment of the acute injury consists of the following:

Extension splint and crutches. The length of time on crutches will depend on the degree of associated meniscal capsular injury.
Cryotherapy with the Cryo-Cuff helps to reduce the swelling and pain.
Physiotherapy to regain range of motion and strength.
Nautilus or gym program to strengthen the muscles with machines and to improve the cardiovascular fitness with steppers and bikes.
Functional brace to stabilize the knee in pivotal motions. Note that Martinek has shown that knee bracing is not required after ACL reconstruction.
Counseling concerning knee friendly sports and activities.
Gradual return to sports as the range of motion and strength improves.
Follow-up evaluation to assess the success of the conservative program.

The nonoperative program for the chronic ACL deficient knee consists of the following:

The use of a functional custom fitted brace, such as the DonJoy Defiance brace.
A progressive strengthening exercise program for the hamstrings and quadriceps conducted in a gym. Cardiovascular conditioning should also be done with bicycling, stair climbing, and similar activities.
Counseling for activity modification to reduce pivoting sports. Knee friendly sports such as biking and cross country skiing should be encouraged, rather than basketball and soccer.

Surgical Indications

The indications for surgical treatment of the ACL tear are the following:

A young competitive pivotal athlete who wants to return to sports.
The failure of a nonoperative program, with persistent pain, swelling, and giving way.
A desire to increase the level of athletic activity without the use of a brace.
A repairable meniscal tear in a young athlete. The meniscus repair has a high failure rate unless the knee is stabilized with an ACL reconstruction.

Frequently Asked Questions About the ACL

Patients will ask many questions about the surgical procedure. The most frequently asked questions, with appropriate responses, are given below.

What Is the ACL?

The ACL is the main crossed ligament in the middle of the knee that connects the femur (thigh bone) with the tibia (shin bone). It controls the rotation of knee and prevents giving out of the knee with pivotal motions of the leg.

Why Should You Have Surgery to Repair the ACL?

You only need to have an ACL reconstruction if you are physically active in pivotal sports such as basketball, volleyball, or soccer. Only approximately 10% of patients who have injured their ACL can return to these sports without an ACL reconstruction. Some patients can use a brace, modify their activities, and resume sports without surgery. The best option for the young, pivotal athlete is to have a reconstruction to prevent episodes of giving way because of ACL laxity. With each reinjury, there is risk of further damage to the meniscus and articular cartilage. The ACL can be reconstructed with fairly predictable results, but the long-term outcome depends on the damage to the meniscus and articular surface. The goal of the ACL reconstruction is to provide a stable knee and prevent further damage to the meniscus and articular cartilage.

Do I Need the Surgery If I Am Not Involved in Pivoting Sports?

The answer is no. The ACL is used only during pivoting motions. Sometimes the giving way sensation may be the result of a torn meniscus that may be repaired with a minor operation. An older, recreational athlete may function fine with activity modification and the use of a brace. Every surgical procedure has a risk benefit, and ACL reconstruction is no exception. If the patient can modify activities to avoid pivotal motions, the knee may function well without surgery.

What If I Have an ACL Tear and I Continue Pivoting Sports?

The patient pursuing this approach will probably suffer giving way episodes, accompanied by pain and swelling. In the long term, this will cause wearing of the inside of the knee (osteoarthritis). The patient who wants to carry on with vigorous pivoting sports should have an operation to reconstruct the knee.

How Does the Physician Know That the ACL Is Completely Torn?

It does not matter whether the ligament is partially or completely torn. If the knee is lax, as can be measured by clinical examination or with the KT-1000 arthrometer, the ACL is not functioning to protect the knee against pivotal motions. The MRI can determine if the ligament is completely torn, but cannot differentiate the degree of laxity.

Is It Possible That More Than the ACL Is Injured?

After the initial injury, there is a 50% chance of damage to the meniscus. In the acute situation, the meniscus tear may be repaired. In the chronic situation, the incidence of meniscal tear is 75%, and the torn portion of the meniscus usually has to be removed.

What Happens to the Knee Joint When the Meniscus Is Removed?

In the long term, the removal of all, or part of the meniscus, is associated with an increased incidence of osteoarthritis.

What Is the Average Time Needed Before the Patient Can Return to Sports After the Surgery?

The answer is four to six months, but sometimes, it may take as long as one year to fully return to a pivotal sport.

How Long Will the Patient Be Out of Work?

It depends entirely on the type of work. If the work involves physical activity, it will take three to four months or until your legs are strong enough. If the work is sedentary, it will probably take two to three weeks.

When Can the Patient Start Driving After Surgery?

Driving can be resumed when weight bearing is comfortable. This usually is sooner when the left knee is involved.

Is Physical Therapy Necessary? How Hard Is It?

Physical therapy is necessary for approximately one to six weeks postoperatively. The therapy goal is to reduce the pain and swelling, regain range of motion, and increase the strength of the muscles. Therapy may have to be modified based on the individual's progress through the weeks of rehabilitation. To view the rehabilitation program, see Chapter 8.

Which Graft Is Better: the Semitendinosus or the Patellar Tendon?

The choice of a graft is almost immaterial. The outcome of the ACL reconstruction depends not so much on the type of graft, but on the technique of placing the graft in the correct position, the fixation of the graft, and the postoperative rehabilitation. Because of the minimum harvest site morbidity, the most common graft used in our sports clinic is the hamstring graft. The patellar tendon graft is used for the athlete who wants to return to sports quickly, for example, at three months. The earlier return to activities is based on the faster healing of the bone-to-bone healing of the patellar tendon graft when compared to the tendon-to-bone healing with the hamstring graft. The latter may take as long as three months to heal. In a recent metaanalysis of the literature comparing the hamstring and patellar tendon grafts, no significant difference in outcome was found. However, the patellar tendon grafts were a little more stable, and the patient was able to return to the same level of sports 18% more often than those who received the hamstring graft.

What About Synthetic Grafts?

Synthetic materials are not routinely used to substitute for the ACL because of the higher incidence of failure. These materials are indicated in special situations, such as multiple ligament injuries or some reoperations.

What About the Allograft?

The allograft is obtained from a cadaver, so a minimal risk of disease transmission exists. In addition, the graft takes longer to incorporate and often has tunnel enlargement as a result. Long-term results have shown more failures with the use of the allograft than with other options.

How Long Does the Patient Have to Use the Special Knee Brace?

After the surgery, the patient will have to use a Zimmer extension splint, or a functional brace for four to six weeks to protect the graft until it heals to the bone. The patient can return to sports four to six months after surgery, but with the brace on. The brace can be discarded a year after the procedure.

How Are the Screws Removed?

Surgery is not required to remove the screws. Because the screws now used are made of a special sugar-type compound, they will dissolve within a couple of years after the surgery.

Is the Surgery a Day Care Procedure?

The answer is yes. The patient will spend just a few hours in the hospital day care recovery room after the surgery.

Does the Giving Way Cause Pain after the Acute Episode?

The answer is yes. It also can cause more damage to the articular surface and the meniscus, thereby leading to later osteoarthritis.

Does the Harvest of the Graft Cause a Problem with the Knee Later On?

The answer is yes. There is some weakness of the hamstrings after removal of the semitendinosus and the gracilis tendons. There is usually no weakness after patellar tendon harvest, but pain around the kneecap is common postoperatively.

Will the Knee Wear Out If the ACL Is Not Fixed?

More damage, or "wearing out," of the articular surface will occur if the knee continues to give way. Giving way should be prevented by activity modification, bracing, or surgical reconstruction. Shelbourne has shown that if the ACL tear is isolated, and there is no meniscal or cartilage damage at the time of the original surgery, the X-ray of the knee will be normal in 97% of the cases. This means that athletes who have a reconstruction and continue to be active can have a normal knee after 10 years.

What Are the Potential Complications of ACL Surgery?

The complications that may occur after ACL reconstruction are those that are related to any surgical procedure such as infection and deep venous phlebitis (i.e., blood clot in the calf). The complications specifically related to the operation are loss of range of motion, anterior knee pain, persistent pain and swelling, and residual ligament laxity because of graft failure. An injury to the nerves or blood vessels after this type of surgery is extremely uncommon.

5
Graft Selection

History

The type of graft that the surgeon chooses for ACL reconstruction has evolved over the past few decades. In the 1970s, Erickson popularized the patellar tendon graft autograft that Jones had originally described in 1960. This became the most popular graft choice for the next three decades. In fact, in a survey of American Academy of Orthopaedic Surgeon members done in 2000, 80% still favored the use of the patellar tendon graft.

In the light of harvest site morbidity and postoperative stiffness associated with the patellar tendon graft, many surgeons began to look at other choices, such as semitendinosus grafts, allografts, and synthetic grafts. Fowler and then Rosenberg popularized the use of the semitendinosus. However, even Fowler was not convinced of the strength of the graft. Then, Kennedy and Fowler developed the ligament augmentation device (LAD) to supplement the semitendinosus graft. Gore-Tex (Flagstaff, AZ), Leeds-Keio, and Dacron (Stryker, Kalamazoo, MI) were choices for an alternative synthetic graft to try to avoid the morbidity of the patellar tendon graft. The initial experience was usually satisfactory, but the results gradually deteriorated with longer follow-up.

Allograft was another choice that avoided the problem of harvest site morbidity. The initial allograft that was sterilized with ethylene oxide had very poor results. Today the freeze-dried, fresh-frozen, and cryopreserved are the most popular methods of preservation of allografts. The allograft has become a popular alternative to the autograft because it reduces the harvest site morbidity and operative time. However, Noyes has reported a 33% failure with the use of allografts for revision ACL reconstruction.

The aggressive postoperative rehabilitation program advocated by Shelbourne in the 1990s greatly diminished the problems associated with the patellar tendon graft. Before that, the patient had to be an athlete just to survive the operation and rehabilitation program. The aggressive program emphasized no immobilization, early weight bearing, and extension exercises.

There was renewed interest in the semitendinosus during the mid-1990s. Biomechanical testing on the multiple-bundle semitendinosus and gracilis grafts demonstrated them to be stronger and stiffer than other options. This knowledge combined with improved fixation devices such as the Endo-button gave surgeons more confidence with no-bone, soft tissue grafts. The Endo-button made the procedure endoscopic, thereby eliminating the need for the second incision.

Fulkerson, Staubli, and others popularized the use of the quadriceps tendon graft. This again reduced the harvest morbidity, especially when only the tendon portion was harvested.

Shelbourne has described the use of the patellar tendon autograft from the opposite knee. He claims that this divides the rehabilitation between two knees and reduces the recovery time. With the contralateral harvest technique, the average return to sports for his patients was four months.

With both the patellar tendon and the semitendinosus added to the list of graft choices, the need for the use of an allograft is minimized.

The latest evolution is to use an interference fit screw to fixate the graft at the tunnel entrance. This produces a graft construct that is strong, short, and stiff. It means that the surgeon now has to learn just one technique for drilling the tunnels and can chose whatever graft he or she wishes: hamstring, patellar tendon, quadriceps tendon, or allograft.

Successful ACL reconstruction depends on a number of factors, including patient selection, surgical technique, postoperative rehabilitation, and associated secondary restraint ligamentous instability. Errors in graft selection, tunnel placement, tensioning, or fixation methods may also lead to graft failure. Comparative studies in the literature show that the outcome is almost the same regardless of the graft choice. The only significant fact from the metaanalysis, as confirmed by Yunes, is that the patellar tendon group had an 18% higher rate of return to sports at the same level. The most important aspect of the operation is to place the tunnels in the correct position. The choice of graft is really incidental. Studies by Aligetti, Marder, and O'Neill show that the only significant differences among the grafts is that the patellar tendon graft has more postoperative kneeling pain.

Evolution in Graft Choice at Carleton Sports Medicine Clinic

The most popular graft in the early 1990s was the patellar tendon graft (Fig. 5.1). With the evolution of the 4-bundle graft and improved fixa-

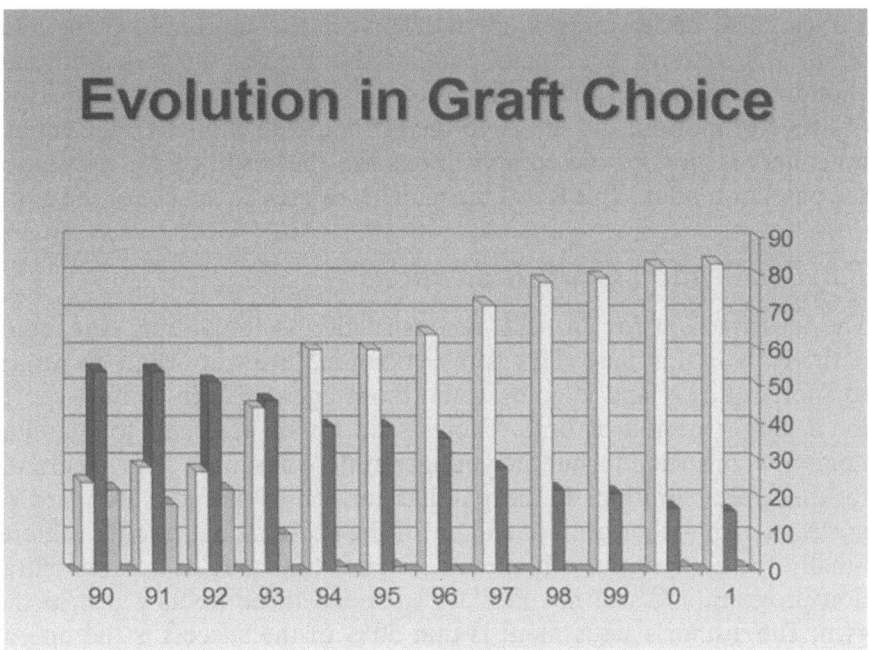

FIGURE 5.1. The evolution of the graft choice. The white bar is the hamstring graft.

tion in the mid-1990s, the hamstring graft became more popular. The swing to hamstring grafts then became largely patient driven. When the patients went to therapy after the initial ACL injury, they saw how easy the rehabilitation was for the hamstring tendon and opted for that graft.

The main choices of graft for ACL reconstruction are the patellar tendon autograft, the semitendinosus autograft, and the central quadriceps tendon, allograft of patellar tendon, Achilles tendon, or tibialis anterior tendon, and the synthetic graft.

Patellar Tendon Graft

The patellar tendon graft was originally described as the gold-standard graft. It is still the most widely used ACL replacement graft (i.e., it is used in approximately 80% of cases), but it is not without problems.

Shelbourne has pushed the envelope further with the patellar tendon graft. He has recently reported on the harvest of the patellar tendon graft from the opposite knee, with an average return to play of four months postoperative.

The advantages of the patellar tendon graft are early bone-to-bone healing at six weeks, consistent size and shape of the graft, and ease of harvest. The disadvantages are the harvest site morbidity of patellar tendonitis, anterior knee pain, patellofemoral joint tightness with late chondromalacia, late patella fracture, late patellar tendon rupture, loss of range of motion, and injury to the infrapatellar branch of the saphenous nerve. Most of the complications are the result of the harvest of the patellar tendon. This is still the main drawback to the use of the graft.

Patellar Tendon Graft Indications

The ideal patient for an ACL reconstruction is the young, elite, competitive, pivotal athlete. This is the young athlete who wants to return to sports quickly and is going to be more aggressive in contact sports for a longer period of time. There is no upper age limit for patellar tendon reconstruction, but the younger athlete has more time to commit to knee rehabilitation. If the patellar tendon is the gold standard of grafts, then this is the graft of choice for the professional, or elite, athlete. Finally, the competitive athlete understands the value of the rehabilitation program and will not hesitate to spend three hours a day in the gym. The author's assessment is that 50% of the success is the operation, and 50% is the rehabilitation program.

Pivoting Activities

The ACL is only required for pivotal athletics. Most nonpivotal athletes can usually cope without an ACL. Cyclists, runners, swimmers, canoeists, and kayakers, for example, can function well in their chosen sport without an intact ACL.

Athletic Lifestyle

This operation should be reserved for the athletic individual. In most activities of daily living the ACL is not essential. If the nonathlete has giving way symptoms, it is probably the result of a torn meniscus and not a torn ACL. The meniscal pathology can be treated arthroscopically, and the patient can continue with the use of a brace as necessary.

Patellar Autograft Disadvantages

Harvest Site Morbidity

The main disadvantage of the patellar tendon graft is the harvest site morbidity. The problems produced by the harvest are patellar tendonitis, quadriceps weakness, persistent tendon defect, patellar fracture, patellar tendon rupture, patellofemoral pain syndrome, patellar entrapment, and arthrofibrosis. The common long-term problem is kneeling pain.

Kneeling Pain

The most common complaint after patellar tendon harvest is kneeling pain. This can be reduced by harvesting through two transverse incisions. This reduces the injury to the infrapatellar branch of the saphenous nerve.

Patellar Tendonitis

Pain at the harvest site will interfere with the rehabilitation program. The strength program may have to be delayed until this settles. The problem is usually resolved in the first year, but it can prevent some high performance athletes from resuming their sport in that first year.

Quadriceps Weakness

The quads weakness may be the result of pain and the inability to participate in a strength program. If significant patellofemoral symptoms develop, the athlete may be unable to exercise the quads.

Persistent Tendon Defect

If the defect is not closed, there may be a persistent defect in the patellar tendon. This results in a weaker tendon.

Patella Entrapment

If the defect is closed too tight, the patella may be entrapped, and patellar infera may result. This will certainly result in patellofemoral pain, because of an increase in patellofemoral joint compression.

Patella Fracture

The fracture may occur during the operation or in the early postoperative period. Intraoperative patella fracture may be the result of the use of osteotomes. If the saw cuts are only 8-mm deep and 25-mm long, and the base is flat to avoid the deep V cut, an intraoperative fracture is rare. The late fractures are produced by the overruns of the saw cuts. The overruns may be prevented by cutting the proximal end in a boat shape.

The left X-ray (Fig. 5.2) shows a displaced transverse patellar fracture, at three months postoperative. The right X-ray (Fig. 5.3) shows the postoperative internal fixation with cannulated AO screws and figure-of-eight wire.

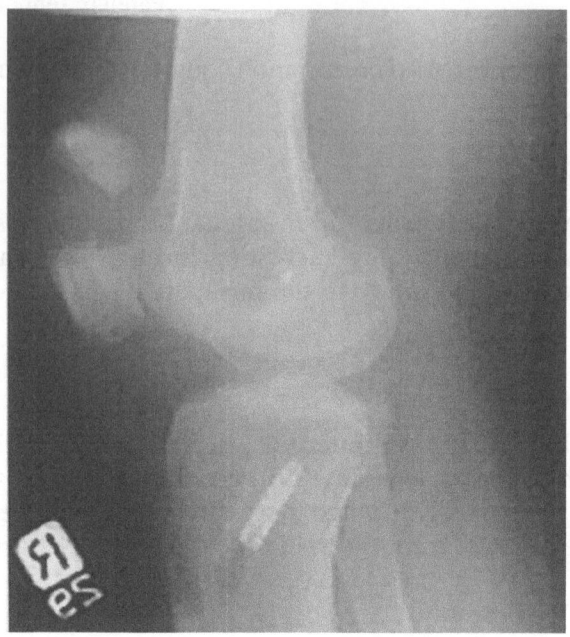

FIGURE 5.2. X-ray of displaced transverse patellar fracture at three months postoperative.

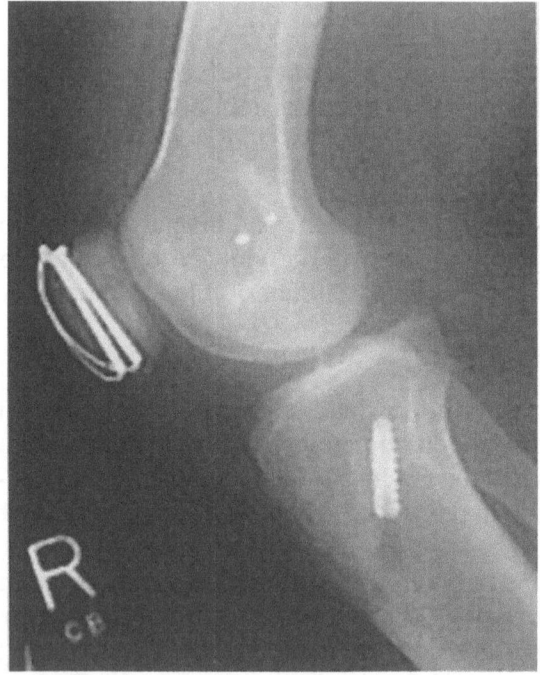

FIGURE 5.3. X-ray of postoperative internal fixation with cannulated AO screws and figure-of-eight wire.

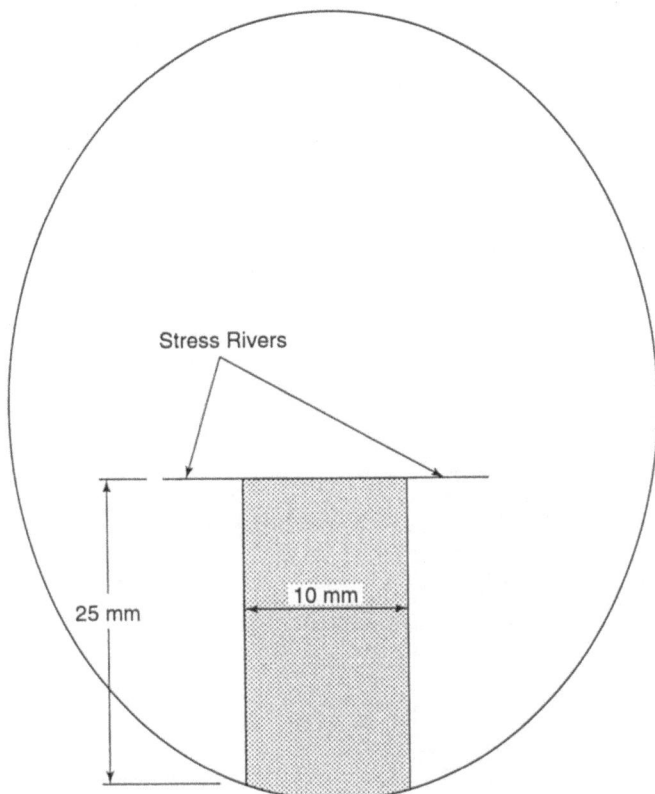

FIGURE 5.4. The method of cutting the patellar bone plug to avoid a late fracture.

The proximal transverse saw cut is critical (Fig. 5.4). The stress risers that go beyond the edge of the bone block should be avoided. An overrun of 2 mm may cause a late transverse patellar fracture. If there are overruns, the burr may be used at the corner to round these cuts. The fracture is usually sustained by muscular contraction. Change to making the proximal cuts boat shaped to prevent the stress risers (Fig. 5.5). The graft is usually cut to this shape to pass into the joint; now it is just cut in that shape before removing it.

Tendon Rupture

This may occur if a very large graft is taken from a small tendon. The standard is a 10-mm graft, measured with a double-bladed knife. The bone blocks are trimmed to 9 mm to make the graft passage easier.

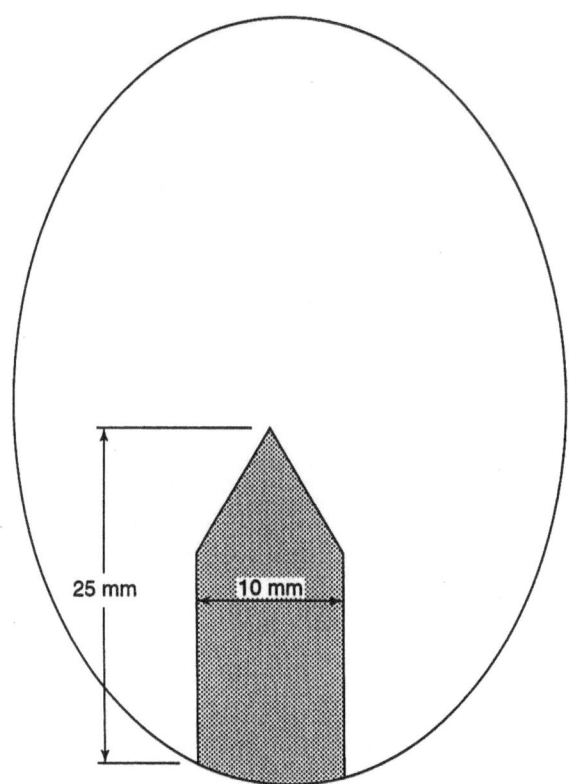

FIGURE 5.5. Boat-shaped proximal cuts.

25 mm

10 mm

Patellofemoral Pain

This topic is controversial in the literature. The older literature reported a high incidence of patellofemoral pain associated with ACL reconstruction. However, most of the disability could be blamed on rehabilitation programs that consisted of immobilization. There is no doubt that some patients will develop pain, some will develop crepitus, and some will have tendonitis, but results have improved with more aggressive rehabilitation programs with early motion and weight bearing. To prevent the patella from being bound down, the patella should be mobilized daily by the physiotherapist.

Arthrofibrosis

This severe problem is rarely seen now in ACL reconstructions. The true condition is idiopathic and is probably the result of fibroblastic proliferation. As a result, very little can be done to prevent it. It may be more common in the patient who forms keloid.

The more common condition of loss of range of motion may be the result of incorrect tunnel placement or postoperative immobilization. In the mid-1980s, a limited range of motion hinge cast (preventing 30° of extension) was used for six weeks postoperatively, thereby causing problems in regaining extension. Many of these cases required arthroscopic debridement (10–18%, in the first year). The loss of extension was almost completely eliminated by changing to an extension splint. The acceptance of aggressive physiotherapy to regain extension eliminated the problem. This problem of postoperative stiffness made the use of a synthetic ligament, with no immobilization, very attractive. The reoperation for loss of range of motion is now very uncommon.

Contraindications to Harvest of the Patellar Tendon

Preexisting Patellofemoral Pain

Is preexisting patellofemoral pain a contraindication to harvesting the patellar tendon? The conventional wisdom is yes; it would not be a wise procedure in this situation. Rather, it is like hitting a sore thumb with a hammer! In the past, when chondromalacia was seen at the time of arthroscopy, the graft choice would be changed to hamstrings.

The Small Patellar Tendon

The harvesting of the central third of the patellar tendon in a small tendon is more theoretical than practical. The advice in a small patient with a tendon width of only 25 mm would be to take a narrower graft of 8 to 9 mm or use another graft source.

Preexisting Osgoode-Schlatters Disease

Shelbourne has reported that a bony ossicle from Osgoode-Schlatters disease is not a contraindication to harvest of the patellar tendon. Because the fragment usually lies within the bony tunnel, this bone may be incorporated into the tendon graft.

Hamstring Grafts

Advantages of Hamstring Grafts

The main advantage of the hamstring graft is the low incidence of harvest site morbidity. After the harvest, the tendon has been shown by MRI to regenerate. The 4-bundle graft is usually 8 mm in diameter, which is a larger cross-sectional area than the patellar tendon.

Disadvantages of Hamstring Grafts

The disadvantage of any autograft is the removal of a normal tissue to reconstruct the ACL. The harvest of the semitendinosus seems to leave the patient with minimal flexion weakness. One study did show some weakness of internal rotation of the tibia after hamstring harvest. Injury to the saphenous nerve is rare and can be avoided with careful technique. The fixation of the graft remains one of the controversial issues.

Issues in Hamstring Grafts

The major issues with the use of hamstring grafts are:

Graft strength.
Graft fixation.
Graft healing.
Donor site morbidity.
Early rehabilitation.
Graft strength and stiffness.

In one of the earlier studies, Noyes reported that one strand of the semi-t was only 70% the strength of the ACL (Fig. 5.6). However, he

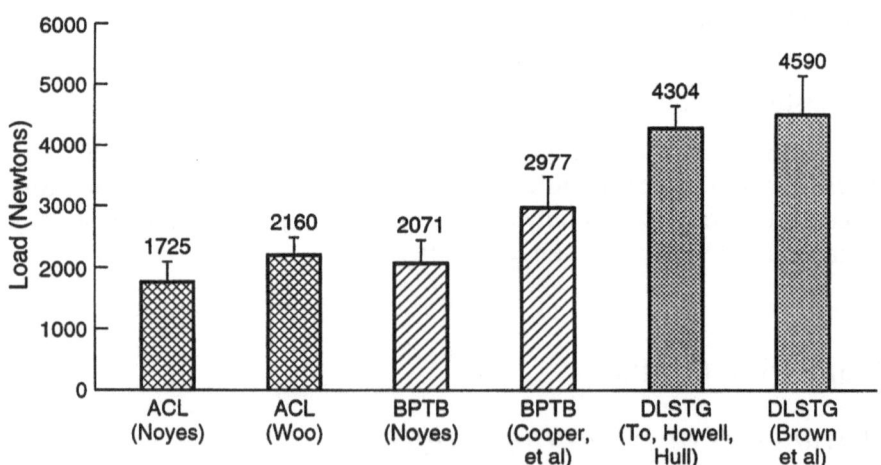

FIGURE 5.6. The ultimate failure load of the normal ACL compared to various grafts.

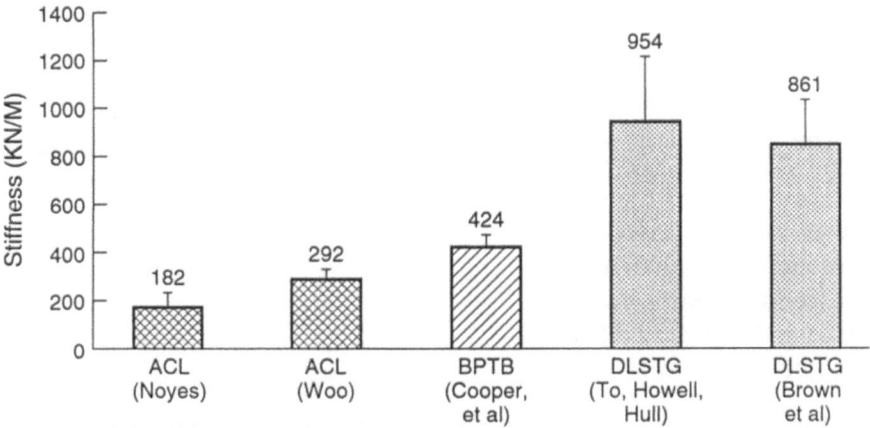

FIGURE 5.7. The composite hamstring graft is twice the strength and stiffness of the native ACL.

compared this to a 15-mm-wide patellar tendon graft that was 125% the strength of the native ACL. This was widely quoted as a reason to use the patellar tendon graft rather than the hamstring. With the advent of the multiple bundles of hamstrings, this graft now has twice the strength of the native ACL (Fig. 5.7). Sepaga later reported that the semitendinosus and gracilis composite graft is equal to an 11-mm patellar tendon graft. Marder and Larson felt that if all the bundles are equally tensioned, the double-looped semi-t and gracilis is 250% the strength of the normal ACL. Hamner, however, emphasized that the strength is only additive if the bundles are equally tensioned.

Soft Tissue Fixation Techniques

There are various techniques for securing the soft tissue to the bony tunnel in ACL reconstruction. Each one has strengths and weaknesses. Pinczewski pioneered the use of the RCI interference fit metal screw for soft tissue fixation. The use of a similar type of bioabsorbable screw that was used in bone tendon bone fixation was a natural evolution. To overcome the weak fixation in poor quality bone, the use of a round pearl, made of PLLA or bone, was developed. This improved the pullout strength by 50%. The Endo-button, popularized by Tom Rosenberg, was improved with the use of a continuous polyester tape. This made the fixation stronger and avoided the problems of tying a secure knot in the tape. The cross-pin fixation has proven to be the strongest, but has a significant fiddle factor to loop the tendons around the post. The Arthrex technique is the easiest to use. Weiler, Caborn, and colleagues have summarized the current concepts of soft tissue fixation.

The estimates of the force on the normal ACL during activities of daily living are as follows:

Level walking: 169N
Ascending stairs: 67N
Descending stairs: 445N
Ascending ramp: 27N
Descending ramp: 93N

It is commonly quoted that a person needs more than 445N pullout strength of the device just to handle the activities of daily living. However, Shelbourne has reported good results with the patellar tendon graft fixed by tying the leader sutures over periosteal buttons (Ethicon, J&J, Boston, MA). This form of fixation has a low failure strength, but is clinically successful.

The gold standard of the interference fit screw fixation of the bone tendon bone, 350 to 750N, has been used to compare the soft tissue fixation.

The pullout strengths also vary from tibia to the femur. The femoral pullout is higher because the tunnel is angled to the graft and the pull is against the screw that is placed endoscopically. In the tibial tunnel, the graft pulls away from the screw in the direct line of the tunnel.

The initial fixation points were at a distance from the normal anatomical fixation of the ACL. The trend has been to move the fixation closer to the internal aperture of the tunnel. This shortening of the intra-articular length has improved the stiffness of the graft.

The pullout strength of bioabsorbable screw can vary widely depending on its composition. The screw fixation has also been shown to be bone quality dependent. These considerations should be taken into account when choosing a femoral fixation device for soft tissue grafts.

Disadvantages

The disadvantages of the hamstring graft are the various methods used to fix the graft to bone, including staples, Endo-button, and interference fit screws. Furthermore, the graft harvest can be difficult, the tendons can be cut off short, and there is a longer time for graft healing to bone, approximately 10 to 12 weeks.

TABLE 5.1. Ultimate load to failure of femoral fixation devices.

Mitek	600N
BioScrew	400N
Endo-button: tape	500N
BioScrew: Endo-pearl	700N
Bone mulch screw	900N
Cross pin	900N
Endo-button with closed loop tape	1300N

Pullout Strengths of Soft Tissue Devices

The fixation of the graft depends on both the tibial and femoral fixation. The rehabilitation protocol should reflect the type of fixation used. All the femoral fixation devices provide reasonable fixation (Table 5.1). The cyclic load is more important than the ultimate load to failure. The interference screw fares worst with cyclic loads.

Interference Fit Screws

The interference fit screw is shown is Figure 5.8.

Advantages

The advantages are as follows:

Quick, familiar, and easy to use.
Direct bone to tendon healing, with Sharpey's fibers at the tunnel aperture.
Less tunnel enlargement.

Disadvantages

The disadvantages are as follows:

Longer graft preparation time.
Bone quality dependent.
Damage to the graft with the screw.
Divergent screw has poor fixation.
Removal of metal screw makes revision difficult.

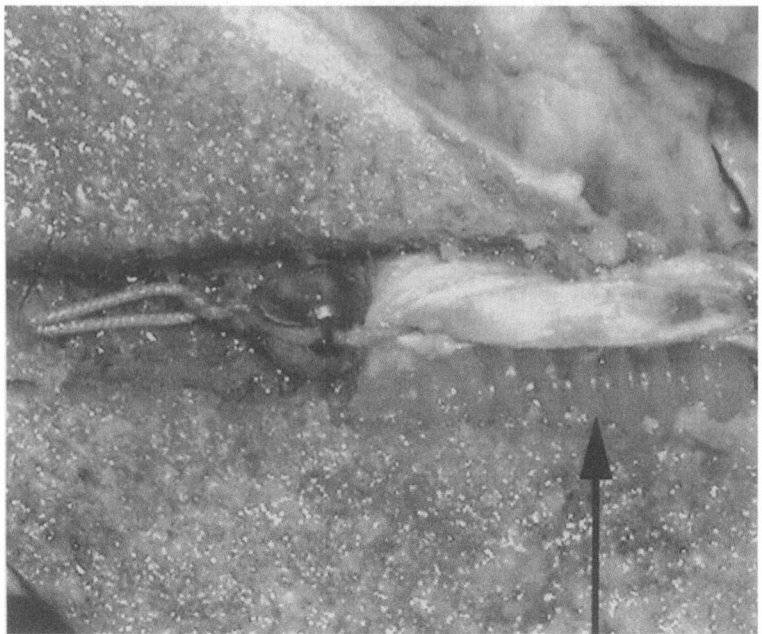

FIGURE 5.8. The interference screw fixation of the soft tissue graft in a cadaver model.

Several refinements have been made to the interference screw technique to increase the pullout strength and cyclic load performance. The end of the graft may be backed up with a round ball of PLLA, the Endo-Pearl (Linvatec, Largo, FL) or bone to abut against the screw and prevent the slippage of the graft under the screw. The tunnels may be dilated or compacted when the bone is osteopenic. A longer screw with a heavy whipstitch in the graft improves pullout strength. The leader sutures from the graft may be tied over a button or post on the tibial side to back up the screw fixation.

Cross-Pin Fixation

The cross-pin fixation is shown in Figure 5.9.

Advantages

The advantages are as follows:

Strongest tested fixation.
May individually tension all bundles of graft.

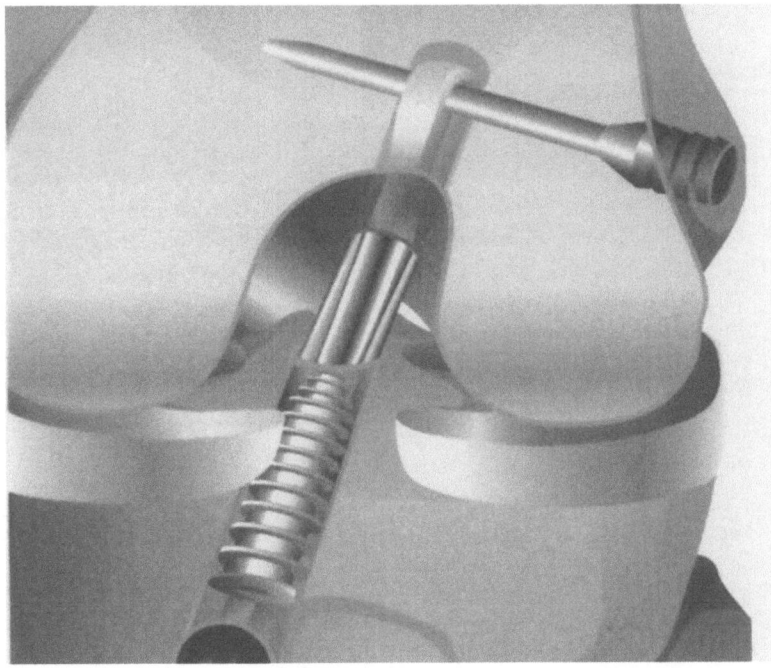

FIGURE 5.9. The Arthrex transfix pin fixation of soft tissues.

Disadvantages

The disadvantages are as follows:

Pin may tilt in soft bone and lose fixation.
Steep learning curve of fiddle factor.
Special guides are required.

Buttons

Buttons are shown in Figure 5.10 and Figure 5.11.

Advantages

The advantages are as follows:

The Endo-button with closed loop tape is strong, if expensive.
The plastic button is cheap, available and easy to do.

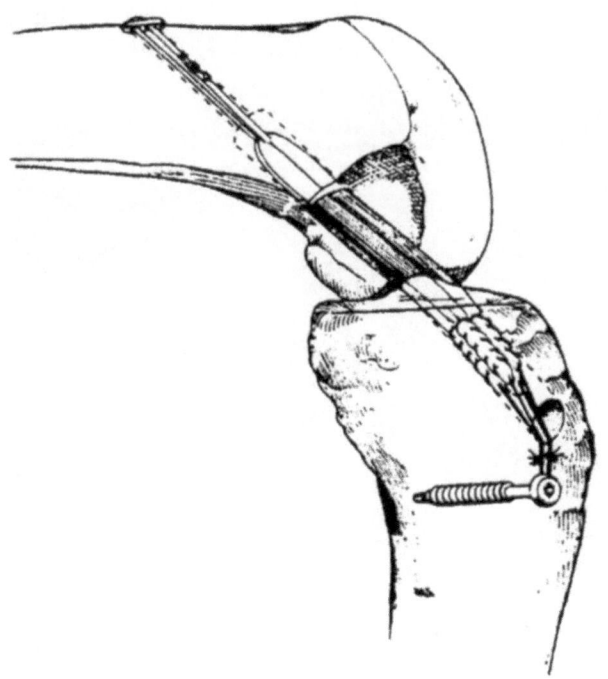

FIGURE 5.10. The Endo-button periosteal cortical femoral fixation of hamstring grafts.

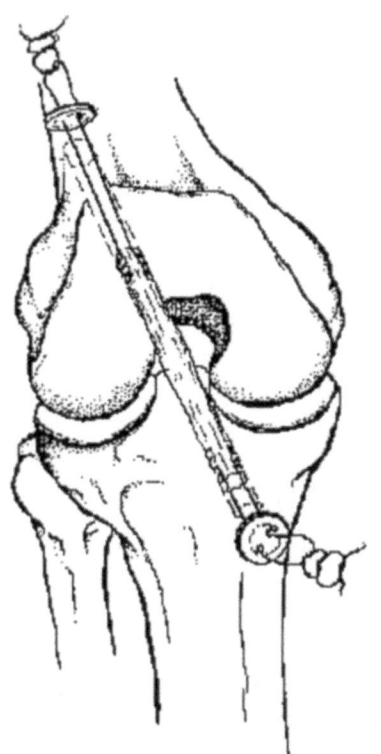

FIGURE 5.11. The periosteal button fixation of soft tissue grafts.

Disadvantages

The disadvantages are as follows:

Fixation site is distant with increase in laxity, with the bungee cord effect.
Increased in tunnel widening.
Plastic button has low pullout strength, dependent on the sutures.

Tibial Fixation

The tibial fixation remains a problem with soft tissue graft fixation. Patients generally do not tolerate metal devices in the subcutaneous area on the front of the tibia. The interference screw gets away from that problem, but has poor performance in cyclic load. The graft tends to slip out from under the screw as the knee is cycled. A backup fixation must be used it the interference screw is used. The Intrafix (Mitek) device uses the interference screw fixation principle, but increases both the ultimate load to failure and the cyclic load performance (Table 5.2).

Considerations

The most important consideration in ACL reconstruction is that the tunnels are put in the correct position. After this, the fixation of the graft is the next most important factor in a satisfactory clinical outcome. The physician should become proficient at one of these techniques. For revi-

TABLE 5.2. Ultimate load to failure of tibial fixation devices.

Single staple	100N
Double staple	500N
Screw post	600N
Button	400N
RCI	300N
BioScrew	400N
BioScrew and button	600N
Intrafix	700N
Screw and washer	800N
Washer Loc	900N

sions, physicians may need to have available another type of fixation to deal with hardware and tunnel expansion.

Tendon-to-Bone Healing

Studies have shown that it takes at least 8 to 12 weeks for soft tissue to heal to bone, as compared to 6 weeks for bone-to-bone healing with the patellar tendon graft. Recent studies have shown that the compression of the tendon in the tunnel with a screw speeds the time of healing, similar to internal compression in bone healing.

Donor Site Morbidity

In 1982, Lipscomb found that after harvest of the semitendinosus only the strength of the hamstrings was 102% and after harvest of both the strength was 98%. Recently, it has been shown that the internal rotation strength is decreased after the harvest of the semitendinosus. The patellofemoral pain incidence has been reported by Aligetti to be 3 to 21% after semitendinosus reconstruction. There are rare reported cases of saphenous nerve injury.

Early Rehabilitation

Prospective randomized studies by Aligetti and Marder have shown that with early and aggressive rehabilitation, there was no difference between the semitendinosus and patellar tendon grafts in stability or final knee rating. This puts to rest the argument as to whether the hamstring graft can withstand early aggressive rehabilitation protocols.

Central Quadriceps Tendon

This graft has been largely ignored in North America over the past decade. An assistant can harvest the graft while the surgeon is doing the notchplasty. It is a large diameter graft, 10×10 mm (Fig. 5.12). The tendon graft is fixed with interference screws for the bone plug and sutures tied over buttons for the tendon end. A bioabsorbable interference screw may be used at the internal aperture of the tunnel to reduce the tendon motion in the tunnel. The quadriceps tendon graft should reduce the need for the allograft or synthetic in revision cases.

FIGURE 5.12. The quadriceps tendon graft.

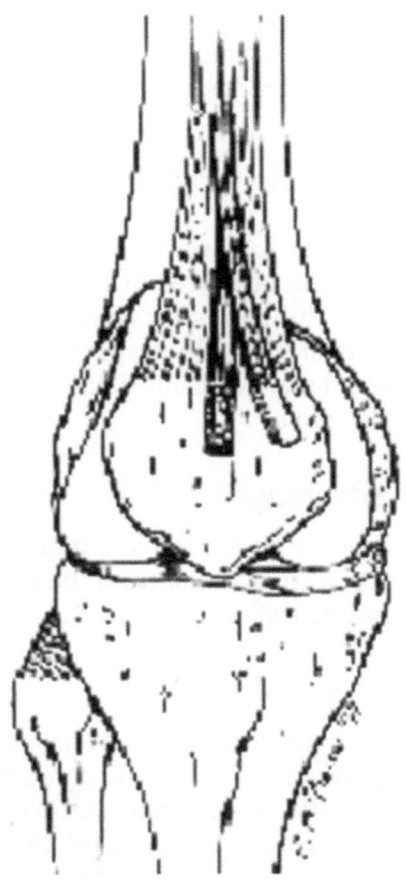

Allografts

Advantages

The allograft has no harvest site morbidity. With no harvest required, the time of the operative procedure is reduced.

Disadvantages

The main objection to the use of the allograft is the risk of disease transmission. Jackson has shown that it takes longer for the graft to incorporate and mature, meaning a longer time until the patient can return to sports. In addition, there is a limited availability of allograft materials. In the literature, Noyes has shown that in long-term follow-up, failure rates increase. In the 1997 survey of the ACL study group by Campell, none of the members used allografts for primary reconstructions.

Synthetic Grafts

The best scenario for the use of the LARS synthetic graft is when the graft can be buried in soft tissue, such as in extra-articular reconstruction. This allows for collagen ingrowth and ensures the long-term viability of the synthetic graft. It will be sure to fail early if it is laid into a joint bare, especially going around tunnel edges, and is unprotected by soft tissue.

Advantages

There is no harvest site morbidity with the use of the synthetic graft. The graft is strong from the time of initial implant. There is no risk of disease transmission.

Disadvantages

The main disadvantage is that all the long-term studies have shown high failure rate. There is the potential for reaction to the graft material with synovitis, as seen with the use of the Gore-Tex graft. With the Gore-Tex graft, there was also the increased risk of late hematogenous joint infection. The results that have been reported with the use of the Gore-Tex graft suggest that it should not be used for ACL reconstruction. Unacceptable failure rates have also been reported with the use of the Stryker Dacron ligament and the Leeds-Keio ligament. The ligament augmentation device was also found to be unnecessary.

6
Hamstring Graft Reconstruction Techniques

Technique of ACL Reconstruction with Semitendinosus

The steps of ACL reconstruction are as follows:

EUA and documentation.
Diagnostic arthroscopy and meniscal repair/meniscectomy.
Graft harvest and preparation.
Stump debridement and notchplasty.
Tibial tunnel.
Femoral tunnel.
Graft passage and fixation.
Final inspection and measurement.

EUA and Documentation

The Lachman test, the pivot-shift test (Fig. 6.1) and the collateral ligament examination should be performed under an anesthetic. The KT-1000 (Fig. 6.2) measurements should also be made and recorded. The criteria for reconstruction is a positive pivot-shift test and a measurement of more than 5 mm in the KT-1000 manual maximum side-to-side comparison.

KT-1000 Measurements, Joint Injection, and Femoral Nerve Block

First confirm which is the correct side. The physician's initials (Fig. 6.3) should be visible on the correct knee. The low profile leg holder is high on the thigh to allow the graft passing wire to penetrate the anterolateral thigh. The tourniquet is placed proximal under the leg holder.

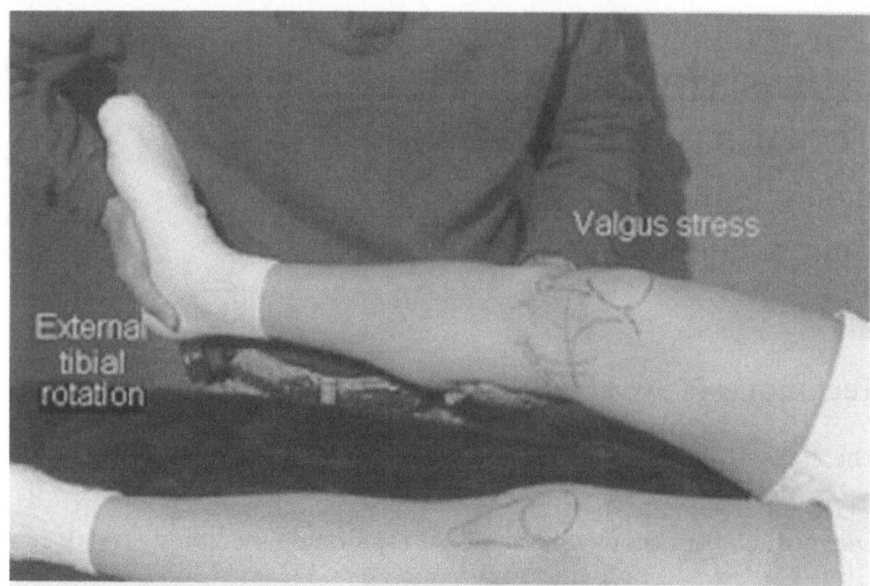

FIGURE 6.1. The pivot-shift test.

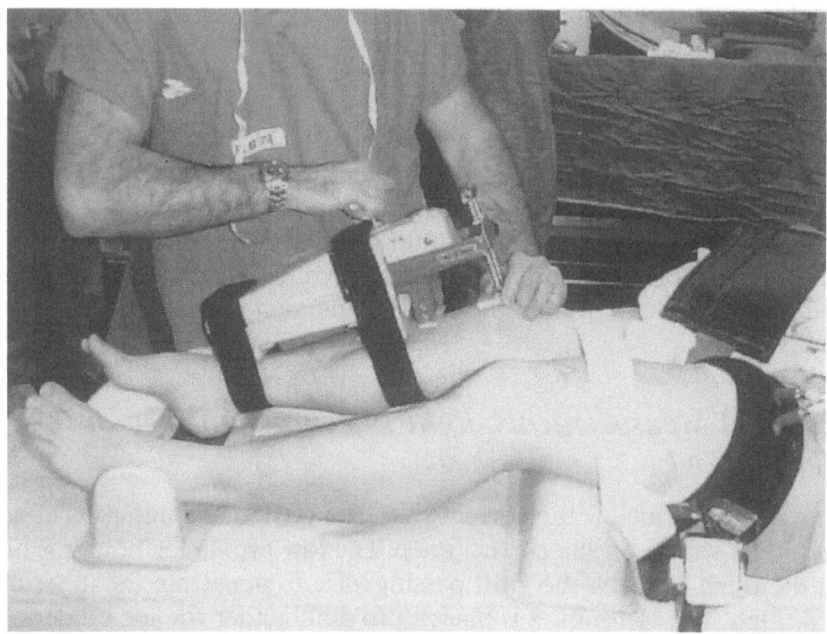

FIGURE 6.2. The KT-1000 arthrometer measurement of the anterior-to-posterior motion of the knee.

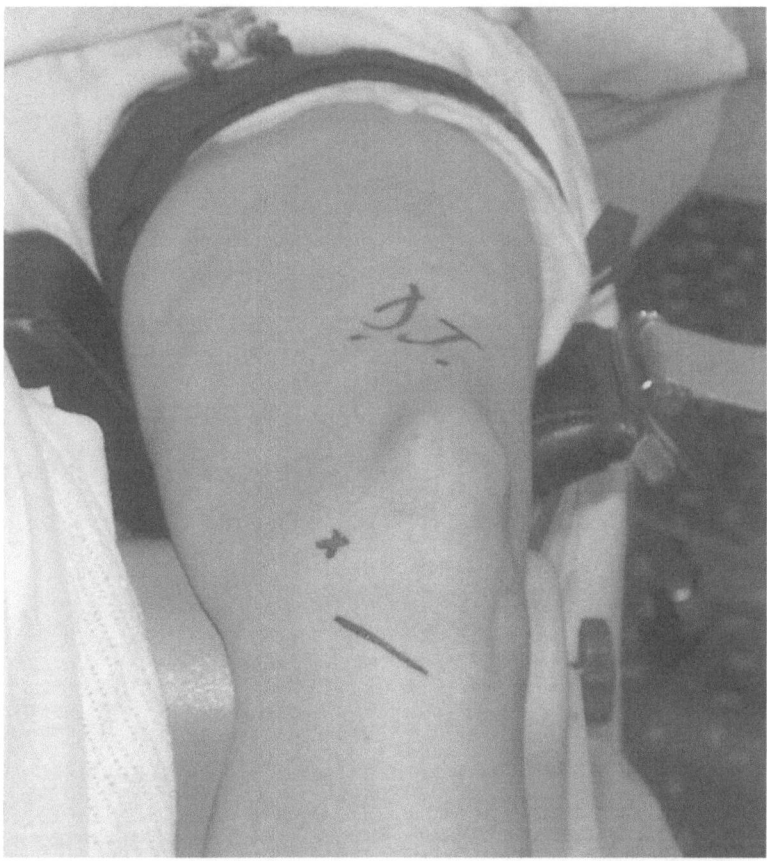

FIGURE 6.3. The setup for ACL reconstruction showing the tourniquet, the leg holder and the marking to determine the correct site for surgery. The incision for the harvest of the tendon is also marked.

Preemptive Pain Management

In a recently published paper, we documented the benefit of the preemptive use of the femoral nerve block, intravenous injections, and local knee injections. The anesthetist uses a peripheral nerve stimulator before the arthroscopy to block the femoral nerve (Fig. 6.4). The dosage is 20 cc of 0.25% bupivacaine with adrenaline. The knee joint and the incisions are injected with 20 cc of bupivacaine 0.25% with epinephrine and 2 mg of morphine. The anesthetist gives 30 mg of Toradol intravenously and 1 gm of Ancef intravenously.

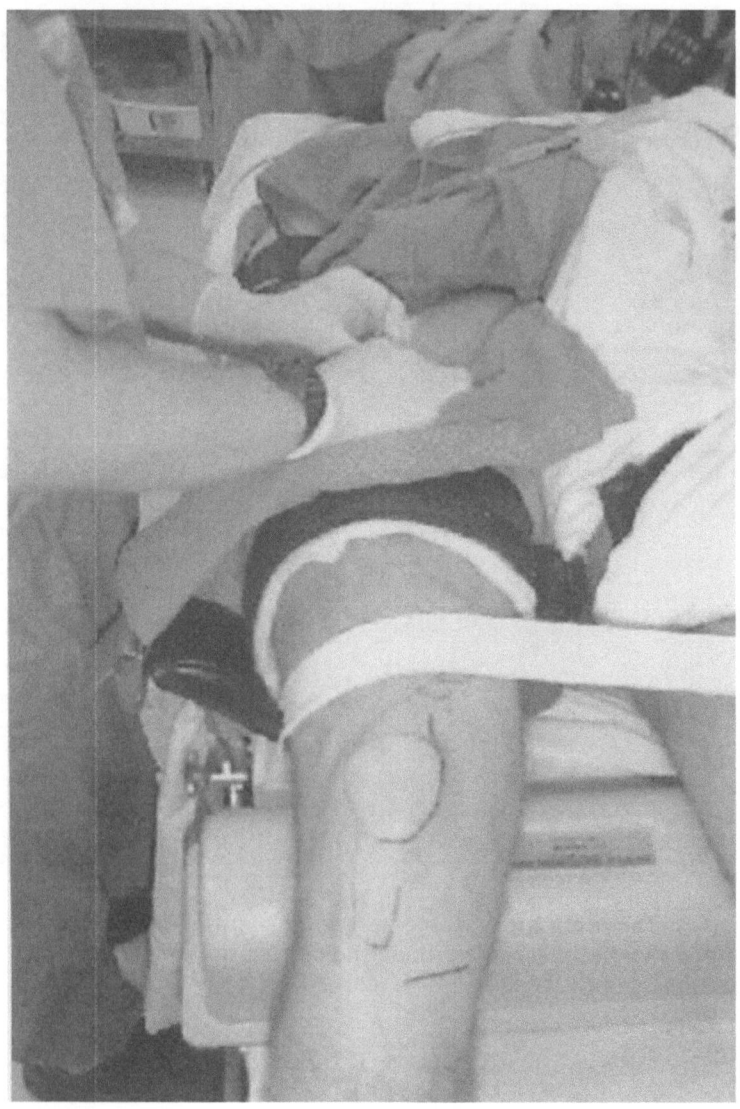

FIGURE 6.4. The femoral nerve block performed with a nerve stimulator.

The physician is now ready to prepare and drape. Use a tourniquet inflated to 300 mm of mercury. The author uses a Linvatec (Largo, FL) fluid pump that works in coordination with the Apex (Linvatec, Largo, FL) driver system for the shaver and burrs to coordinate the flow level. The leg is flexed over the side of the bed.

Diagnostic Arthroscopy and Meniscal Repair/Meniscectomy

The portals must be accurately placed to visualize all aspects of the knee (Fig. 6.5). The high lateral portal, at the corner of the patellar tendon and the patella, is the first portal to establish. The medial portal may be identified with an 18-guage needle before it is cut with the knife (Fig. 6.6).

The "W" maneuver initially scans the entire knee (Fig. 6.7). The order of the examination is as follows:

1. Suprapatellar pouch. Examine the synovium and look for loose bodies.

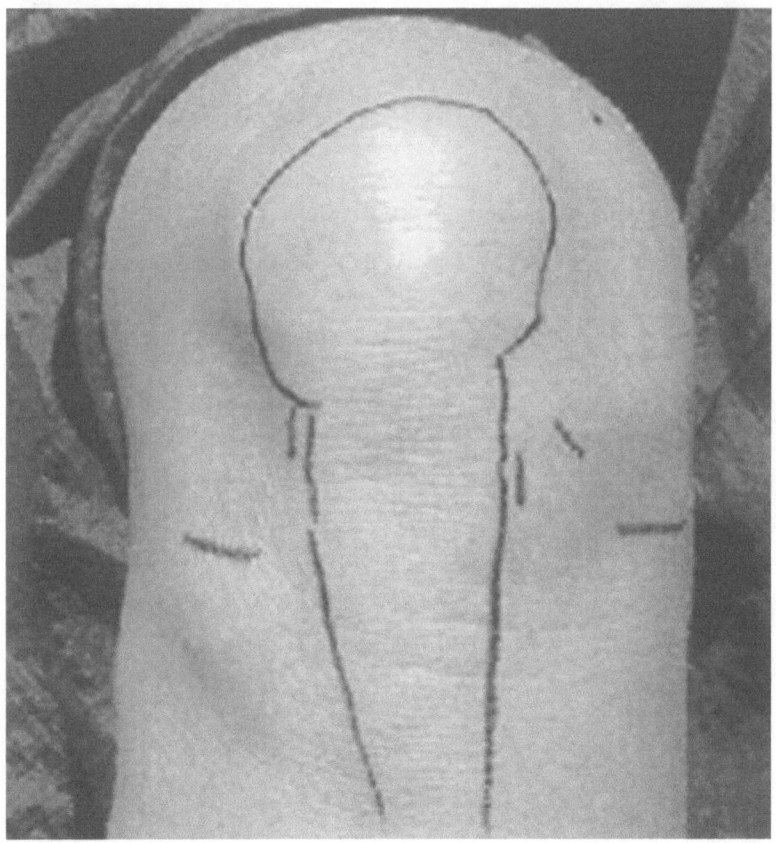

FIGURE 6.5. The anteromedial, anterolateral and the accessory medial portals for ACL reconstruction.

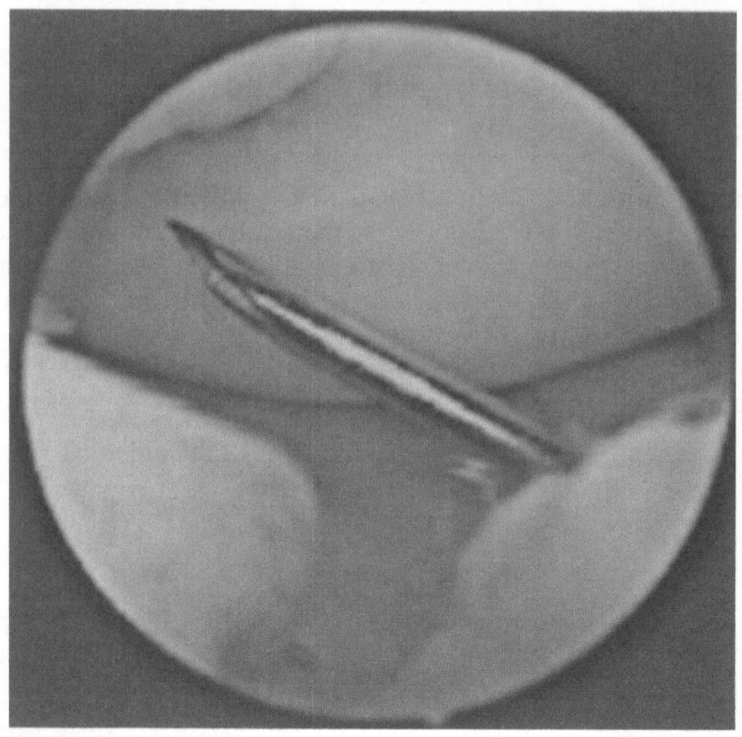

FIGURE 6.6. The localization of the anteromedial portal with an 18-gauge needle while viewing from the high anterolateral portal.

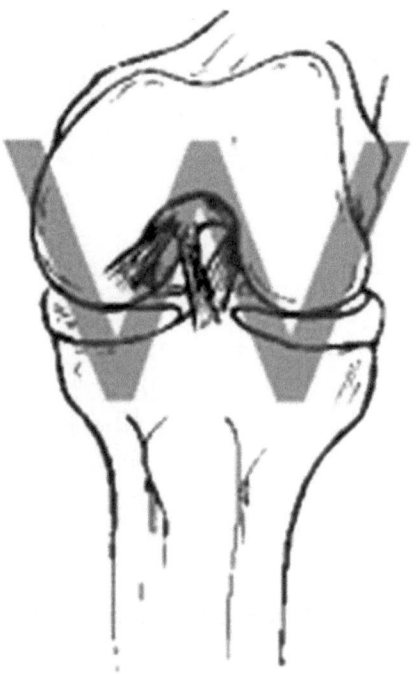

FIGURE 6.7. The "W" maneuver to view the entire joint.

2. Patella and femoral trochlea. Examine the articular cartilage. The medial aspect is inspected for a plica.
3. Medial gutter. Inspect the synovium and look for loose bodies.
4. Medial compartment. Examine the articular surface of the femur and tibia and probe the meniscus with a hook.
5. Intercondylar notch. Inspect the ACL, PCL, and synovium
6. Lateral compartment. Examine the articular surface of the femur and tibia and probe the meniscus with a hook.
7. Lateral gutter. Inspect the synovium and popliteus tunnel and look for loose bodies.

If there is any doubt about the diagnosis or the type of graft, the diagnostic arthroscopy should be done before the graft harvest. The video on the CD illustrates this technique, as well as the inside view of the "W" arthroscopy as described in Chapter 2. The ACL must be carefully examined. The degree of tear must be assessed. The conventional wisdom is that a tear of more than 50% should be reconstructed. But a partial tear, one of less than 50%, may have to be reconstructed with a semitendinosus. If the tear is partial, with a negative pivot shift, this patient should be treated conservatively.

The portals (Fig. 6.5) must be made in the correct position. If there is no meniscal pathology detected on the first diagnostic survey, then the anteromedial portal may be made low to insert the femoral fixation screw. If meniscal repair is required, then the normal medial portal is made, and a second medial accessory low medial portal, to insert the femoral interference screw, will have to be made.

A complete diagnostic arthroscopy should be performed before any meniscal work is done. This ensures that the physician will not forget the lateral compartment if a lot of time is required to perform meniscal repair on the medial side. Asses the entire joint and plan the operative work. In young patients, every attempt should be made to repair the meniscus rather than resect it. The long-term results of reconstruction are more related to the state of the meniscus than the stability.

Indications

First of all, who is a candidate for meniscal repair? The algorithm for meniscal repair should consider the following factors.

Location

The ideal type of meniscal tear to consider repairing is the peripheral tear. This is also referred to as the red on red tear, indicating the degree of vascularity. This tear is amenable only to suture repair. Most commonly the tear is in the red on white region, which also has an acceptable successful repair rate when bioabsorbable devices are used.

Morphology of the Tear

- Size: The short tear of 1 to 2 cm has a better successful repair rate.
- Appearance: The vertical longitudinal tear is ideal for repair. Do not consider repairing degenerative horizontal cleavage tears or flap tears.
- Patient factors.

Noncompliant patients should not be considered for repair.

The younger patient has a higher success rate. The older patient often has the type of degenerative tear that is nonrepairable.
The rehabilitation must be modified to avoid flexion in the immediate postoperative period.
Fifty percent of ACL tears are associated with meniscal tears.

In summary, the best candidate for meniscal repair is the young compliant patient with a 2-cm long peripheral longitudinal meniscal tear.

The Technique of the Repair of a Bucket-Handle Tear of the Meniscus

Step 1: The Diagnosis of the Bucket-Handle Tear

Figure 6.8 shows a longitudinal tear of the meniscus that has displaced into the intercondylar notch. There may be a lot of synovium and fat pad that needs to be removed with a shaver in order to visualize the meniscus.

Figure 6.8 is the diagrammatic representation of a large displaced bucket-handle tear of the meniscus. Figure 6.9 is the arthroscopic view. Often the first view will be a "white out." There is so much synovium and the large displaced tear, that nothing can be seen on the medial side except synovium. In a young patient, this tear should be repaired if possible. The physician should look over the displaced fragment to assess the size of the remaining rim to determine if it is suitable for repair.

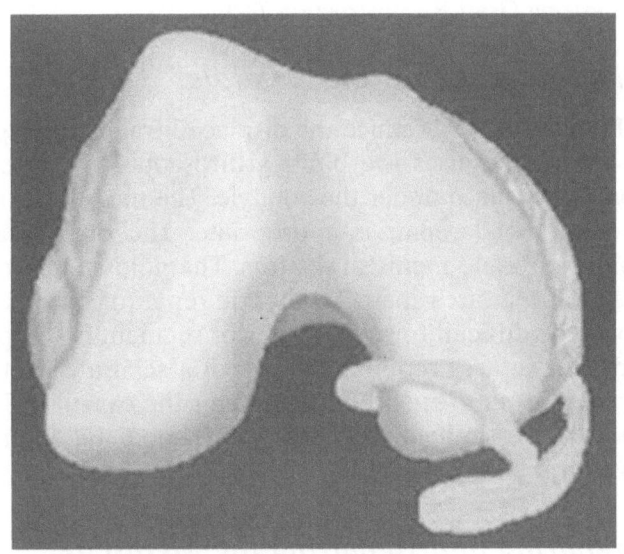

FIGURE 6.8. Diagram of a bucket-handle tear.

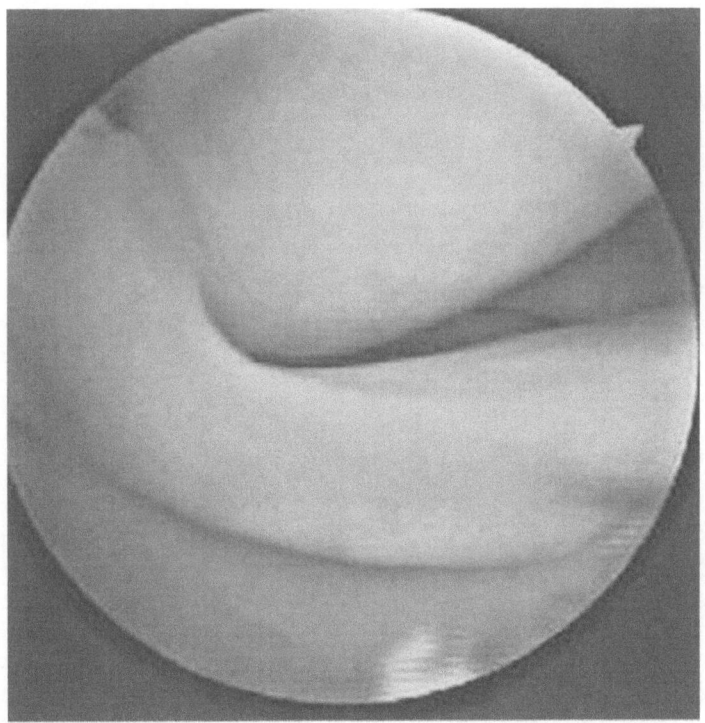

FIGURE 6.9. The arthroscopic view of a displaced bucket-handle tear of the medial meniscus of the right knee.

Step 2: The Reduction of the "Handle"

First, the physician should reduce the displaced fragment (Fig. 6.10 and Fig. 6.11). The author uses the blunt arthroscope trocar to push the meniscus back into place under the condyle. The next decision is which technique of meniscal repair is appropriate. The options are suture repair or bioabsorbable meniscal fixators. The gold standard of repair is considered to be suture repair. The hybrid repair of sutures anteriorly and fixators in the difficult to reach posterior segment is acceptable. The use of inside out sutures requires the use of a separate posterior incision to retrieve the sutures and tie them over the capsule. The incision avoids injury to the saphenous nerve on the medial side and the peroneal nerve on the lateral side.

Step 3: Preparing and Repairing the Meniscus

The tear should be initially probed to determine if it is suitable for repair. The edges of the tear should be débrided of fibrous tissue with a rasp or a small shaver (Fig. 6.12). The meniscus should be rasped to

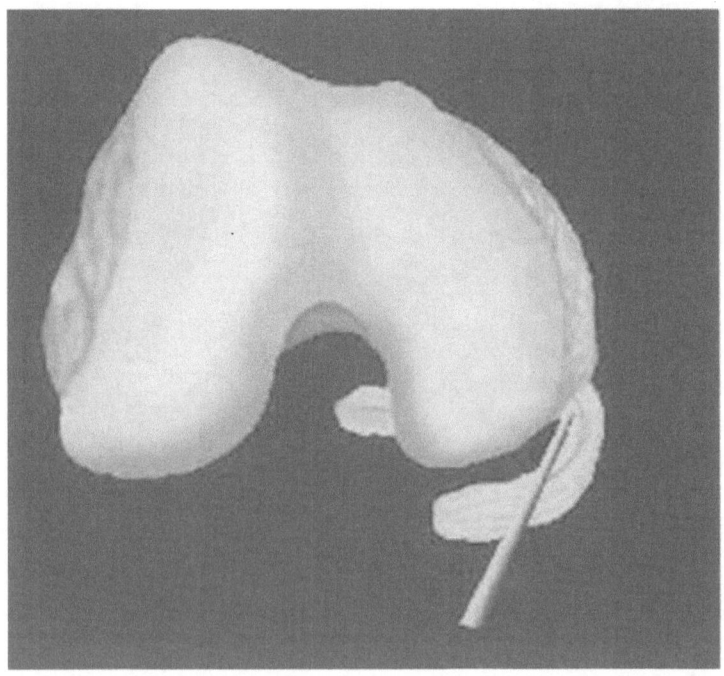

FIGURE 6.10. The reduction of the handle of the tear.

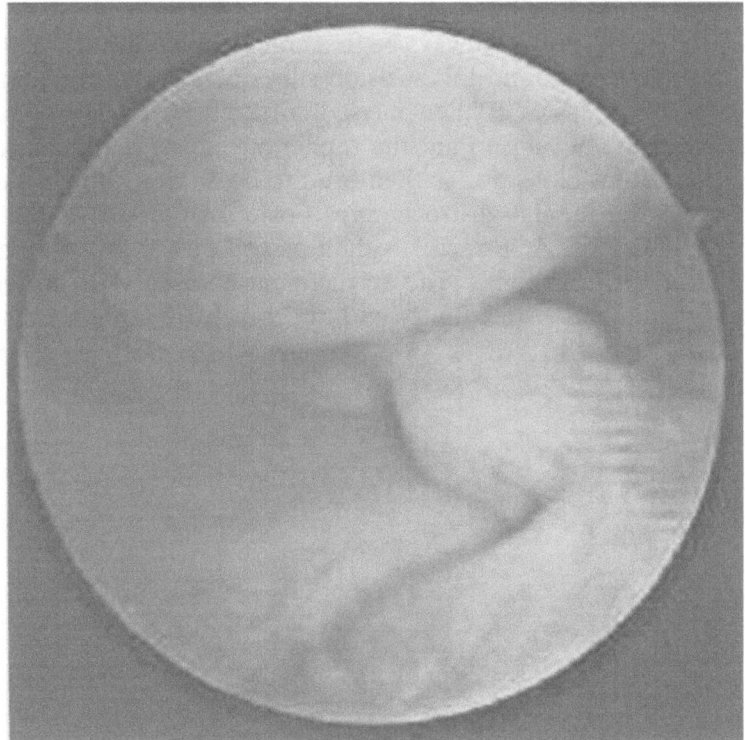

FIGURE 6.11. The arthroscopic appearance of the reduced bucket-handle tear.

stimulate bleeding. Pavlovich has described the technique of stimulation of the meniscal synovial border with electrocautery. The principle is to lightly "burn" the synovium to stimulate a healing response.

The monopolar electrode can be used to stimulate the synovium at the tear. Zhang demonstrated that the meniscus and the rim may be trephinated to produce vascular access channels. The sutures and the bioabsorbable devices must be placed accurately to reduce the tear and hold it until it is healed. The common approach with a large bucket-handle tear is to use sutures in the middle segment to reduce and hold the bucket tear and then use the bioabsorbable devices in the difficult-to-access posterior horn region.

Step 4: The Posteromedial Incision

The next step is to create a posteromedial or posterolateral incision (Fig. 6.13). On the medial side, with the knee at 90° of flexion, this technique is a 3 to 6 cm incision placed just posterior to the medial collateral ligament extending distally from the joint line. As the trajectory of the zone-specific needles will always be in a craniocaudal direction, there is little indication to extend this incision superiorly above the joint line. The presartorial fascia is then incised sufficiently to allow posterior retraction of the pes anserinus; the saphenous nerve may be retracted posteriorly. Blunt dissection is then used to come down upon the joint capsule and the medial gastrocnemius posteriorly and the semimembranosus anteriorly. A retractor is then placed posterior to the medial head of the gastrocnemius. The retractor is necessary to protect the assistant from needle stick injury and to protect the saphenous nerve.

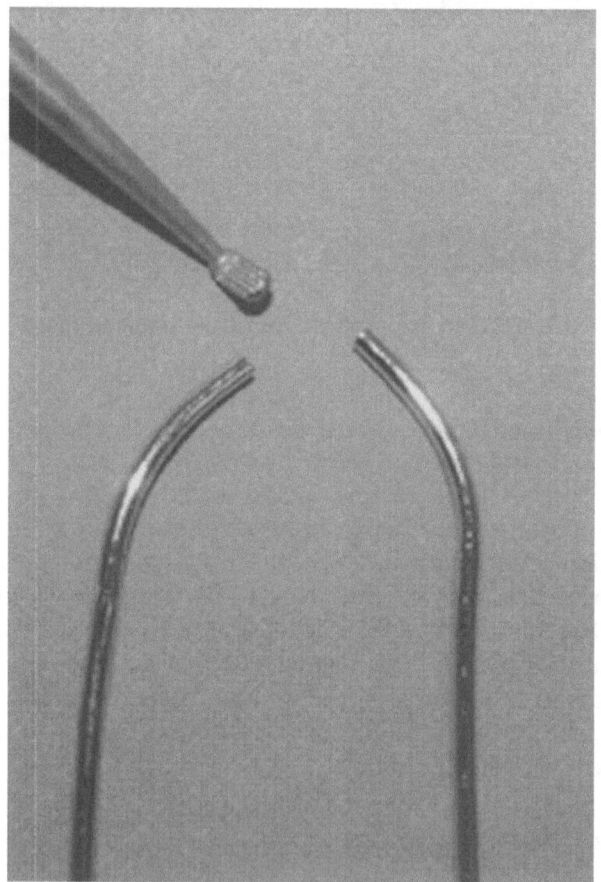

FIGURE 6.12. The rasp for preparing the meniscal tear and the cannulas for inserting the needles.

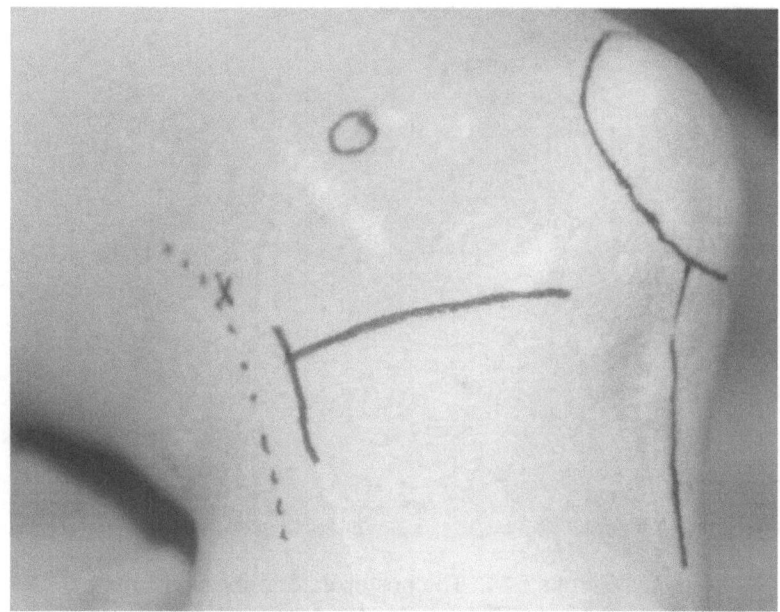

FIGURE 6.13. The posterior medial incision.

Step 5: The Posterolateral Incision

On the lateral side, with the knee at 90° of flexion, an incision may be made posterior to the lateral collateral ligament, again extending 3 cm distal from the joint line (Fig. 6.14). This incision can then be continued with blunt dissection passing between the anterior aspect of the biceps femoris and the posterior aspect of the iliotibial band. The dissection proceeds bluntly, anterior to the lateral head of the gastrocnemius, the arcuate complex, and the capsule. A retractor may then be introduced to protect the neurovascular bundle and the assistant during meniscal repair. The peroneal nerve is traveling just medial to the biceps femoris at this level, where it may be vulnerable if the incision is carried too far proximally or overzealous retraction occurs. Distally to the joint line, the peroneal nerve is protected by posterior retraction of the lateral head of the gastrocnemius.

The Medial Repair: Knee Positioning

The repair of the medial meniscus is performed with the knee in 15° to 45° of extension depending on the location of the tear. The goal of knee positioning is to enable meniscal repair by placing tension on the MCL to visualize the posterior segment of the meniscus.

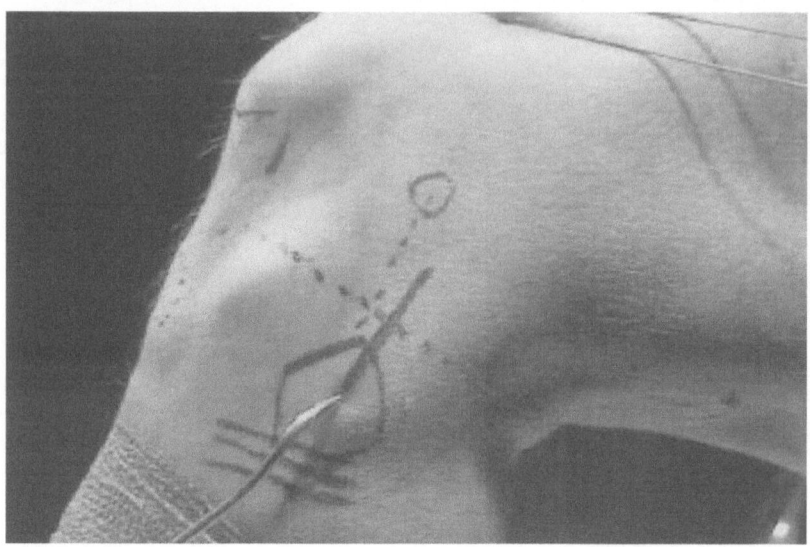

FIGURE 6.14. The posterolateral incision.

The Lateral Repair: Knee Positioning

The lateral meniscus is often repaired in the figure four position, with the knee flexed up on the contralateral ankle with between 45° and 60° of knee flexion. Increased flexion in this manner allows both for increased needle retrieval space by relaxing the gastrocnemius and applying a varus force on the knee. This position also allows for the peroneal nerve to drop further posteriorly, where it is less likely to become stretched. On the lateral side it is occasionally necessary to repair the meniscus to the popliteal tendon to stabilize a posterolateral meniscal tear. Although nonanatomic, this procedure can add substantial stability to a repair.

The Repair: Passing the Sutures

The zone-specific set includes six cannulae, which are 2.7 mm in diameter (Fig. 6.15). Each set includes two cannulae with curves corresponding to the anterior, middle, and posterior zones of the meniscus. The cannulae are labeled for the direction in which they curve. In a variety of circumstances, either a left or a right cannula could be more appropriate for a given knee. The cannulae each have a 15° curve upward, which allows the cannulae to be apposed against the meniscus in the joint and allows the needle to be passed parallel to the joint line from slightly elevated portals. The shapes of the cannulae allow placement of the device around the tibial spines and femoral condyles for needle passage.

The most frequent technique employed involves protruding the needle 2 mm from the tip of the cannulae. A valgus or varus load may be added to the knee at this point to open the compartment of the knee. The needle can then be used to spear the peripheral part of the meniscus and reduce it into position. The needle can then be passed across the tear and retrieved from the incision. The needle should be advanced slowly at 5 mm increments. This will enable the needle to be caught by the retractor tool placed posteriorly. This will serve to protect the neurovascular bundle posteriorly, allow easy retrieval of the needle by the assistant and finally will minimize the opportunity for needle stick

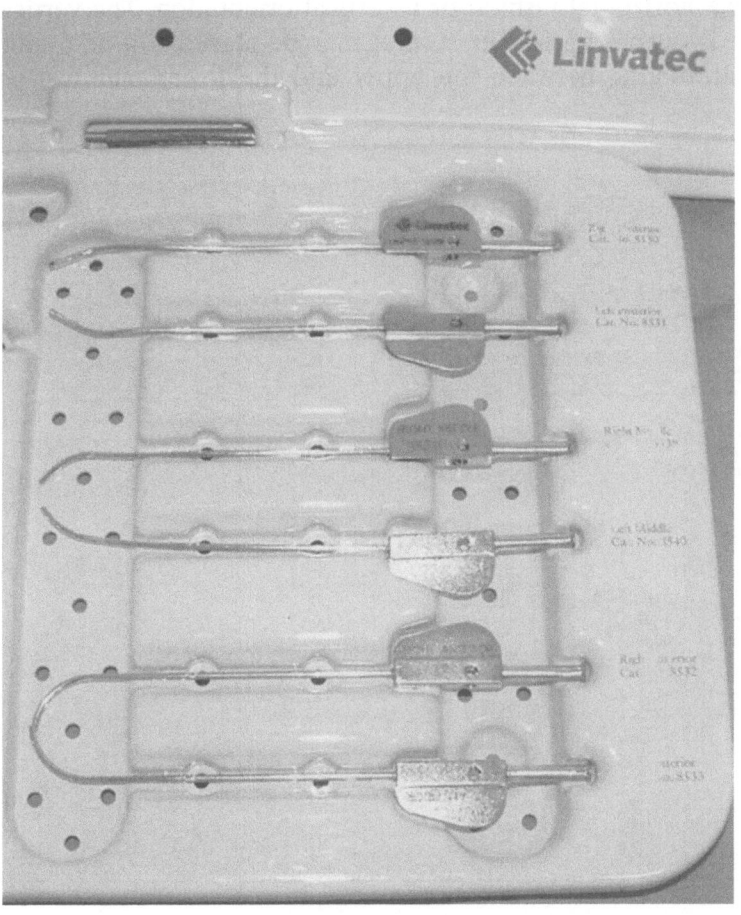

FIGURE 6.15. The zone-specific set of suture passing cannulas.

injuries on the part of the assistant who is retrieving the sutures. For more posterolateral repairs knee flexion of close to 90° may be required in the figure-four position, with or without additional varus (elevation of the ankle).

The sutures are stronger if placed in a vertical loop orientation (Fig. 6.16 and Fig. 6.17). Tension is then placed on the suture to prevent it from kinking in the cannula. The cannula is readjusted to enable placement of a vertical mattress suture and the second stitch is passed. The stitches are made from 2–0 nonabsorbable material, such as Ethibond, and is attached to a 0.24-in. diameter 10-in. needle.

Tears are routinely repaired with the scope in the ipsilateral portal and the cannula coming in from the contralateral portal (Fig. 6.18). Although accessory portals are not routinely needed, they may be used to assist with positioning of the cannulae. Sutures may be placed in either a horizontal fashion or a vertical orientation. The vertical loop suture is the strongest. The sutures may be placed at 4- to 5-mm intervals alternating between the upper and the lower meniscal surfaces

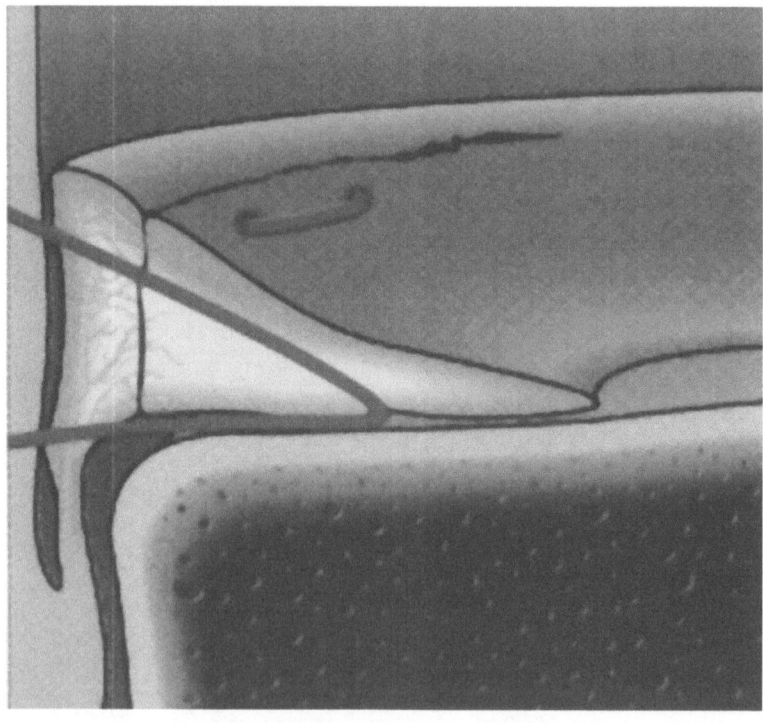

FIGURE 6.16. The loop vertical suture placed under the meniscus with the horizontal loop placed above the meniscus.

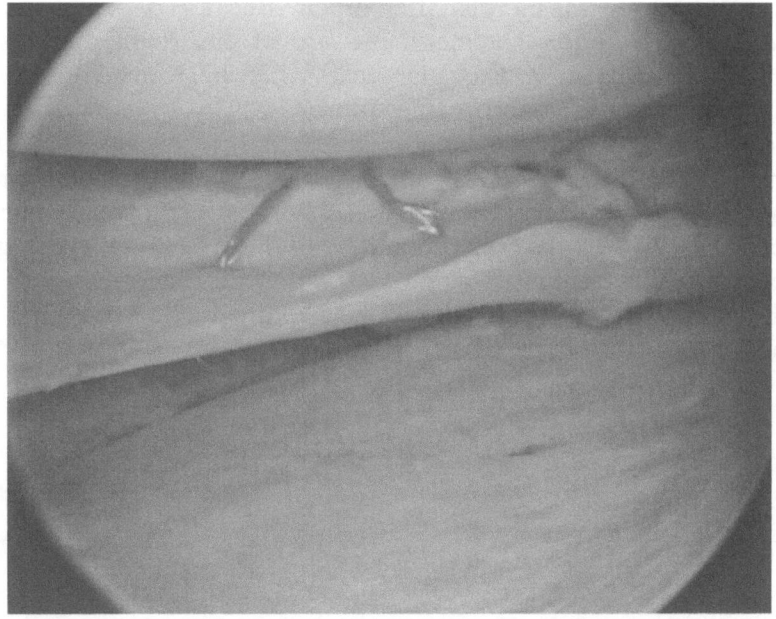

FIGURE 6.17. The vertical loop sutures placed on top of the meniscus.

(Fig. 6.19). If ACL reconstruction is done, the sutures are tightened so that the repair can be verified. The sutures are usually tied after the completion of the meniscal repair and are then tied sequentially over the knee capsule.

Cannon believes that the risk-benefit ratio should discourage the placement of sutures posterior to 1cm from the posterocentral insertion of the posterior horn of the menisci. He believes that the suturing anterior to this point should provide enough strength to reduce and hold the meniscus. Working posterior to this places undue difficulty on the procedure and unnecessary risk to the neurovascular bundle. This has become the major benefit of the hybrid repair, using the sutures for the easy to access mid-portion and the bioabsorbable fixators for the difficult to access posterior region.

Results of Zone-Specific Repair

Rosenberg and his colleagues have evaluated the type of suture used for repair. This group found that the use of nonabsorbable sutures did not abrade or damage the articular cartilage on second look arthroscopy. Further, the group established that in many cases these sutures broke several months after repair. Because of these findings, Rosenberg does not recommend the use of absorbable sutures for routine meniscal tears. Capsular tears that heal quickly may be amenable to the use of absorbable sutures.

Brown et al. stated that 92% of meniscal tears with a rim of less than 4mm had clinically successful outcomes using the signs of meniscal pathology return to sport and the lack of radiographic changes as outcome measures. Several other studies have also reported good success with this technique.

The gold standard for results can be identified by a series that uses second-look arthroscopy as an outcome measure. Rosenberg et al.

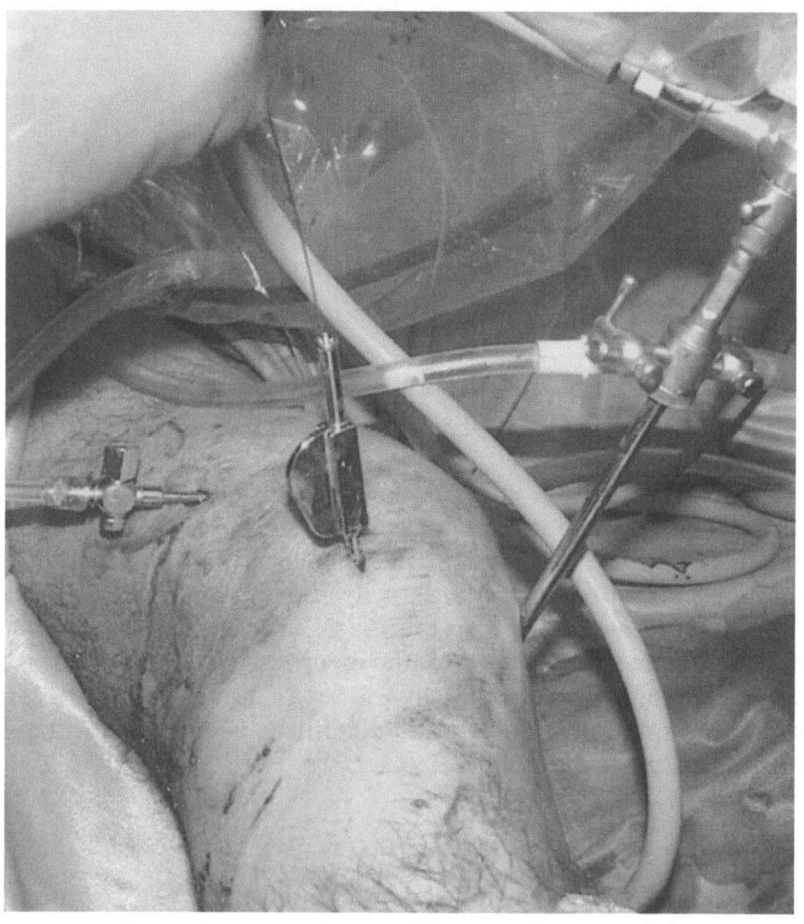

FIGURE 6.18. The cannula is placed in the contralateral portal, while viewing from the ipsilateral portal.

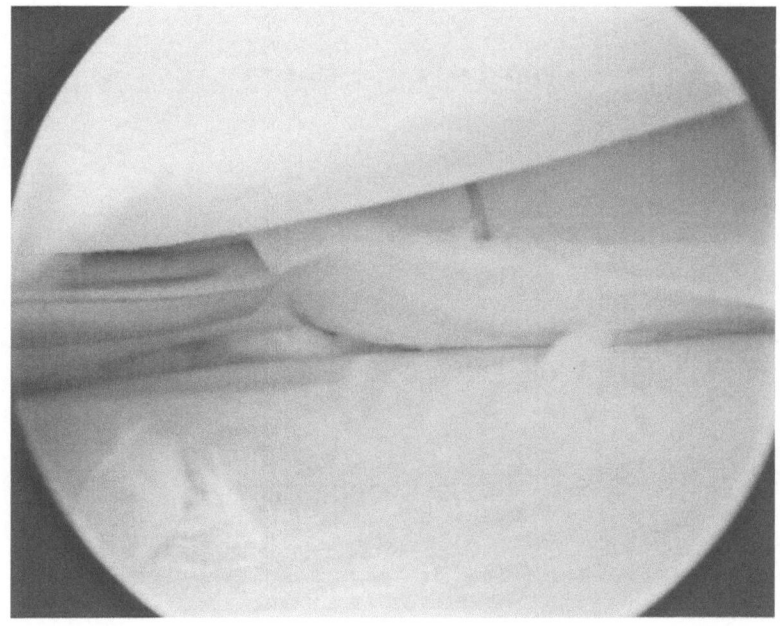

FIGURE 6.19. The completed suture repair with over- and undersutures.

reviewed a series where 24 out of 29 repairs had healed by three months, with the other 5 patients described by his group as partially healed. In the latter group 4 out of 5 of the knees were ACL deficient at the time of repair and second-look arthroscopy.

The Technique of the BioStinger Insertion

The appropriate length of BioStinger (Linvatec, Largo, FL) selected, is usually 13 mm, and loaded on the cannulated wire of the delivery unit (Fig. 6.20). The cannula is placed against the meniscus and 2 mm of cannulated wire is delivered into the torn fragment (Fig. 6.21). The fragment is then reduced to the peripheral rim.

When the torn fragment is reduced, the cannulated wire is advanced into the rim using the slider bar on the side of the device (Fig. 6.22). The BioStinger is inserted into the meniscus by depressing the handle on the end. The meniscus can be felt to ratchet into the meniscus (Fig. 6.23).

To prevent the cannulated wire from bending, firm pressure must be exerted on the cannula to keep this against the meniscus. The cannula is backed up 5 mm, and the head of the BioStinger inspected to be sure

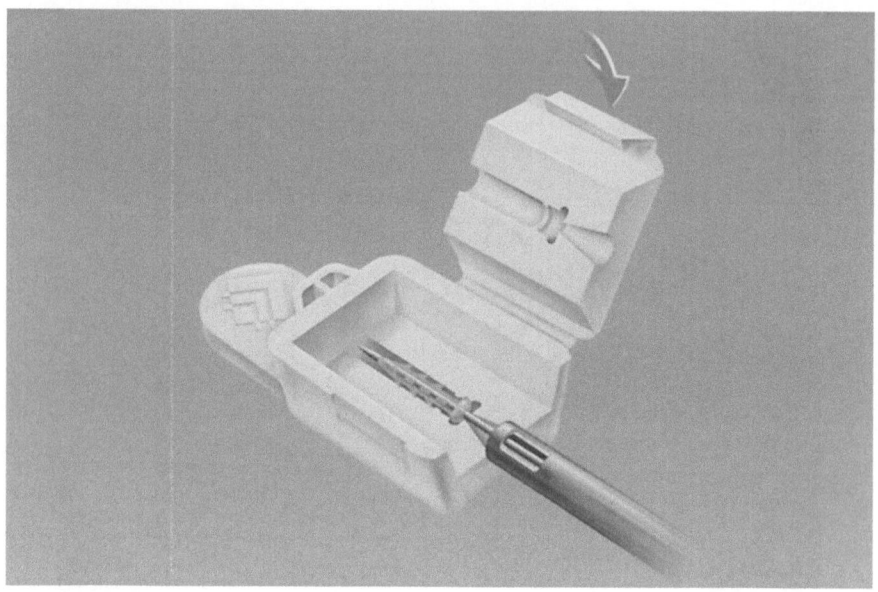

FIGURE 6.20. Loading the BioStinger from the plastic box.

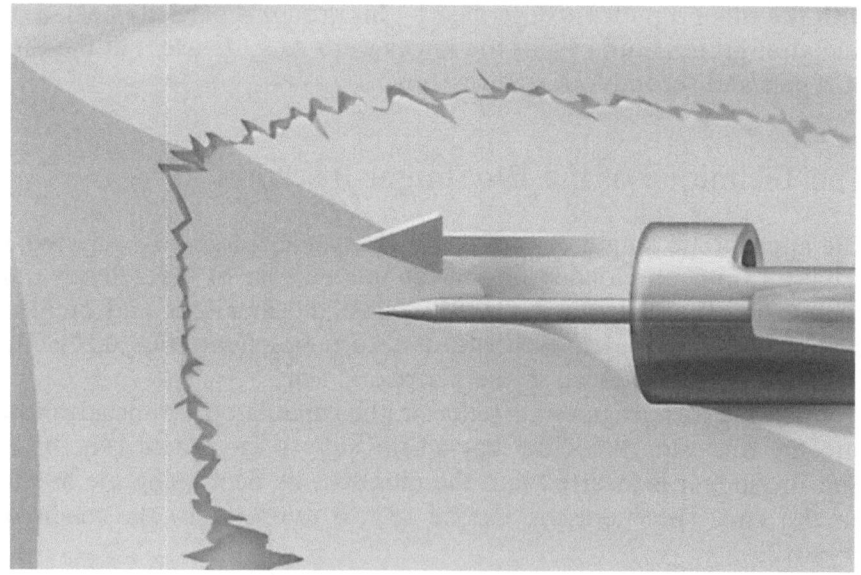

FIGURE 6.21. The initial insertion of the guide wire into the meniscus.

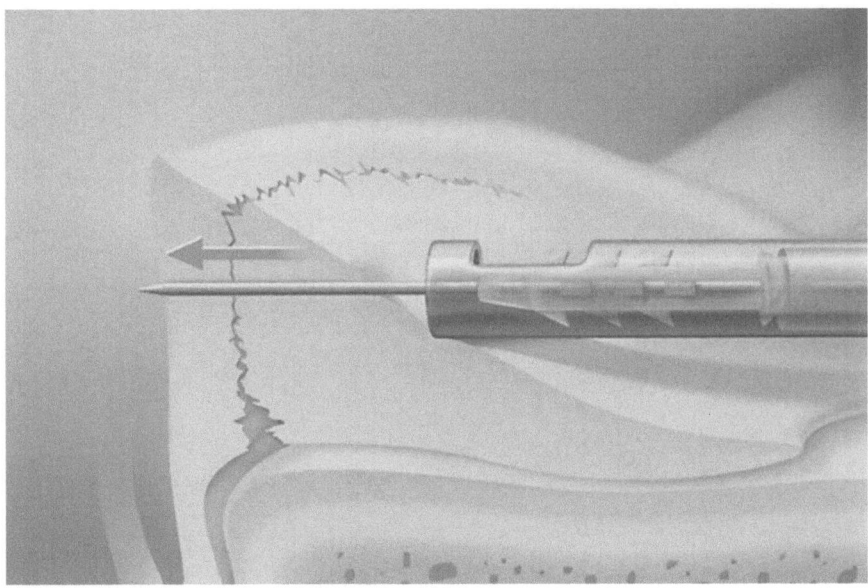

FIGURE 6.22. The advancement of the guide wire across the meniscus tear.

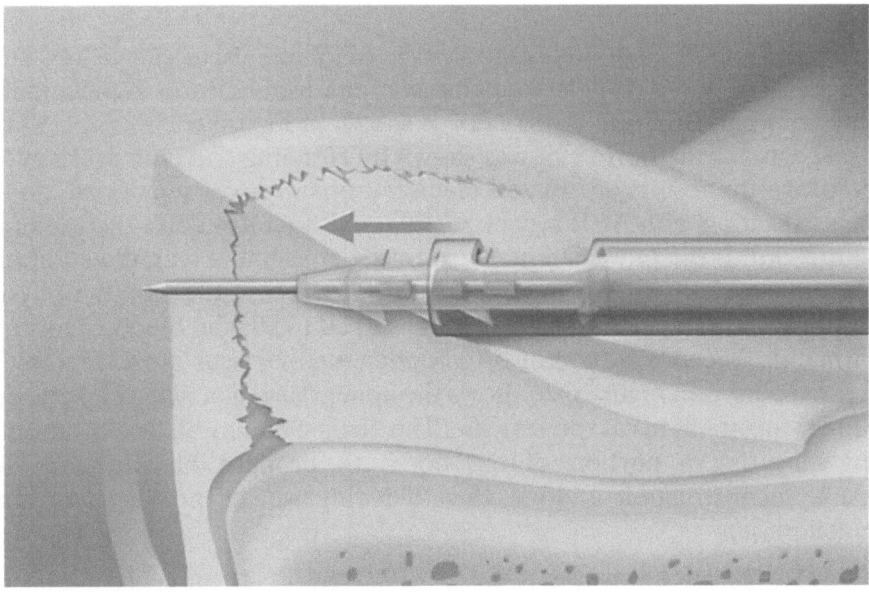

FIGURE 6.23. The BioStinger is driven across the tear by depressing the handle of the delivery device.

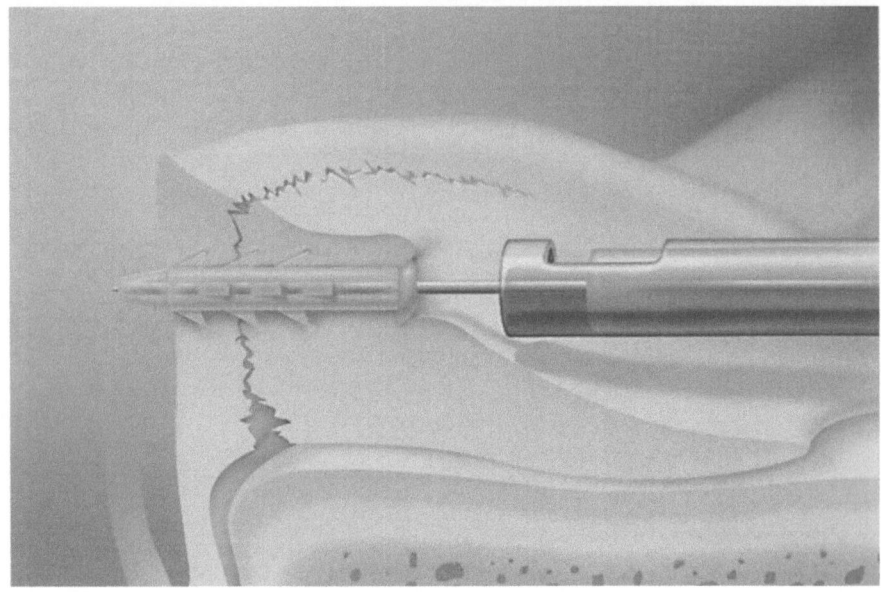

FIGURE 6.24. The BioStinger must be countersunk under the surface of the meniscus.

that it is countersunk under the surface of the meniscus (Fig. 6.24). The appearance of the completed meniscal repair using sutures in the middle segment and BioStinger posterior is shown in Figure 6.25.

The use of the fibrin clot was shown by Henning and later Jackson to improve the results of isolated meniscal repairs. Most repairs are done in association with ACL reconstruction and do not require the use of a fibrin clot. If the physician needs to repair an isolated tear, the addition of a fibrin clot will improve the results. To prepare the clot, the physician will need a glass syringe and a glass rod to stir the blood to form a firm clot. The clot is then inserted under the meniscus at the meniscus synovial border. Figure 6.26 shows the appearance of a fibrin clot placed under the meniscus at the tear site. The fibrin clot may also be produced by curetting a portion of the notch to produce bleeding. If the ACL reconstruction is done, then bleeding will be produced by the notchplasty.

Clinical Results

Peter Kurzweil reported the following results at the Arthroscopy Association of North America (AANA) fall course in San Diego:

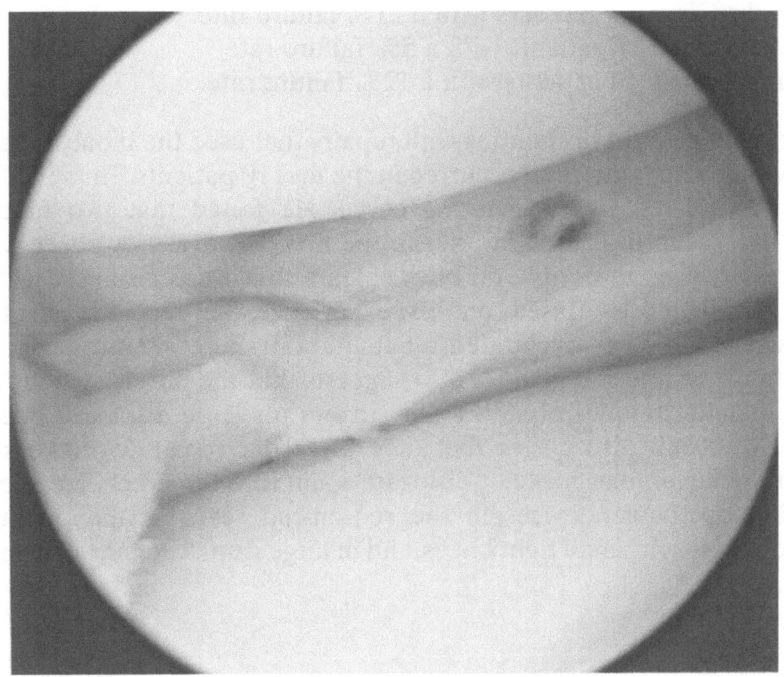

FIGURE 6.25. The completed hybrid repair using sutures and BioStingers.

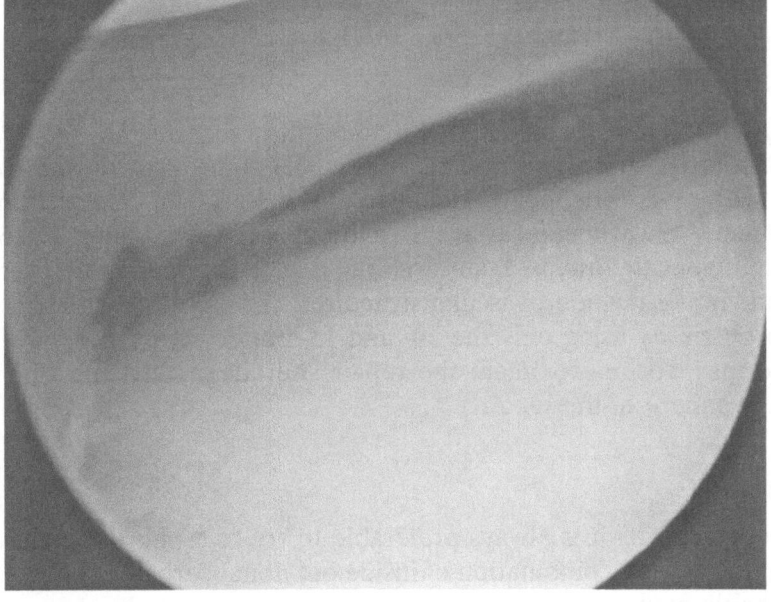

FIGURE 6.26. The fibrin clot placed under the meniscus.

Albrecht-Olsen: 34 patients with a 21% failure rate.
Saul Schrieber: 37 patients with a 5% failure rate.
Peter Kurzweil: 40 patients with a 12% failure rate.

Kurzweil discussed his failures with repairs that used the bioabsorbable arrow. The five failures all occurred in the first 10 patients. Thus, the failures are related to the learning curve. He found that two failures were the result of flexion injuries in the first 3 to 5 weeks. Three were the result of large peripheral bucket tears that were displaced at the time of diagnosis. Based on his experience, he recommends that there should be no accelerated rehabilitation; therefore, no flexion or squatting for four months. He also suggests that the physician combine the repair techniques of suture and arrows for large displaced bucket tears. Kurzweil also cycles the knee after the repair to make sure that the bucket tear does not dislocate again into the notch. He avoids the bioabsorbable devices in the red-on-red tears, in the popliteal tendon region, in small tight knees, and in large displaced bucket-handle tears.

Summary

Meniscus repair in a suitable patient with the appropriate tear is efficacious. The use of the bioabsorbable devices should be used judiciously and in large tears in combination with sutures.

Complications with the Use of the Bioabsorbable Fixators

The use of bioabsorbable fixators may result in fixators that break and become loose in the joint. This may necessitate an arthroscopy to remove the loose fragments. The head of the device may be prominent and damage the articular surface. To avoid this, the device must be countersunk under the meniscal surface. The device may penetrate posteriorly and injure the neurovascular structures. The physician should avoid this problem by using only the 10- and 13-mm devices. Otherwise, the device may not approximate the repair site adequately, and this can result in failure of the repair.

Summary

In young patients it is always preferable to try to repair the meniscus. The author uses a combination of inside out nonabsorbable sutures and absorbable meniscal arrows. He uses the arrows in the hard-to-access region of the posterior horn.

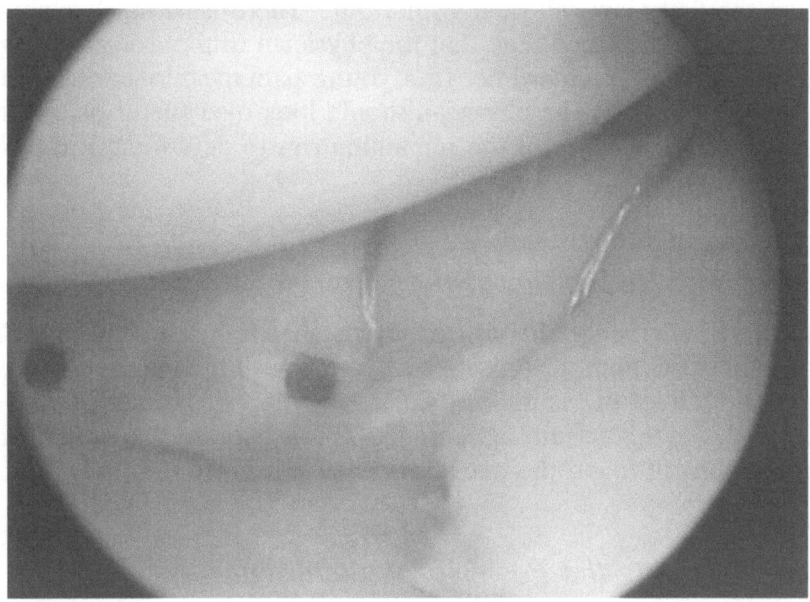

FIGURE 6.27. The arthroscopic view of a hybrid repair.

The combination of vertical sutures in the middle of the meniscus, and bioabsorbable arrows in the posterior region is shown in Figure 6.27. The video on the CD includes a demonstration of the inside out, zone-specific technique of meniscus repair.

The Technique of the Excision of a Bucket-Handle Tear of the Meniscus

Some of the preparation is the same for this procedure, as for the previous procedure. They are repeated here for the sake of completeness.

Step 1: The Diagnosis of the Bucket-Handle Tear

Figure 6.8 shows a longitudinal tear of the meniscus that has displaced into the intercondylar notch. There may be a lot of synovium and fat pad that needs to be removed with a shaver in order to visualize the meniscus.

Figure 6.8 is the diagrammatic representation of a large displaced bucket-handle tear of the meniscus. Figure 6.9 is the arthroscopic view.

Often the first view will be a "white out." There is so much synovium and the large displaced tear, that the physician cannot see anything on the medial side except white. In a young patient, this tear should be repaired if possible. The physician should look over the displaced fragment to assess the size of the remaining rim to determine if it is suitable for repair.

Step 2: The Reduction of the "Handle"

First, the physician should reduce the displaced fragment (Fig. 6.10). The author uses the blunt arthroscope trocar to push the meniscus back. In Figure 6.11, a lot of the anteromedial synovium was removed with the shaver to give this "clean" appearance. This is necessary to see the anterior attachment to cut the bucket handle clean from the rim.

Step 3: Cutting the Posterior Attachment

The posterior attachment is divided first. If the anterior attachment were cut first, the main fragment might displace into the posterior compartment, necessitating a posterior portal to remove it.

Step 4: Insert the Scissors

The scissors are inserted through the medial portal, while visualizing through the anterolateral portal (Fig. 6.28). The torn fragment is cut loose.

To cut the anterior attachment, the scissors are brought in through the anteromedial portal (Fig. 6.29 and Fig. 6.30). The handle can usually be cut from the rim through this portal. If not, the scope is placed in the anteromedial portal and the scissors brought through the anterolateral portal.

Step 5: Removing the Fragment from the Joint

A grasping instrument is used to remove the loose fragment (Fig. 6.31 and Fig. 6.32). Sometimes, it is better to leave a small strand still attached so that the fragment does not migrate around the joint. It is also better to grasp the fragment on the end, so it comes out of the portal easily. If the physician grasps it in the middle, it must fold over and is harder to remove through a small portal.

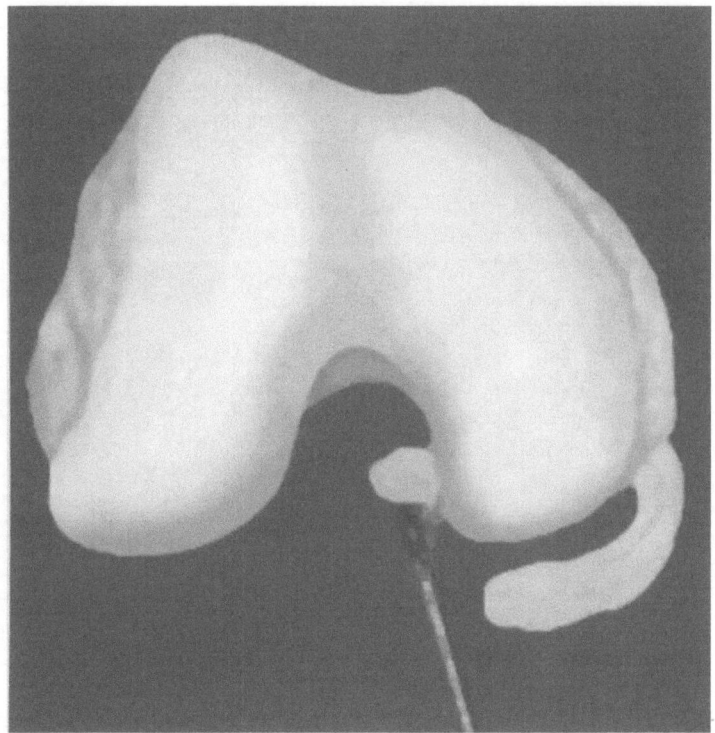

FIGURE 6.28. Cutting the posterior horn attachment of the medial meniscus.

Harvest of the Hamstring Graft

Skin Incision

An oblique 3-cm skin incision is made over the pes anserine (Fig. 6.33). This should start 1 cm medial to the tibial tubercle and head postero-medial. It should be 5 cm below the joint line. The physician should plan to harvest the graft and drill the tibial tunnel through this incision. Then, incise the subcutaneous fat and strip the pes with a sponge.

Exposure of the Tendon

The physician should identify the superior border of the pes and incise the fascia. Then, continue the incision medially, in a hockey stick fashion, down the tibia to remove the attachment site. A kocher is used to traction this flap. Look for the most inferior tendon, the semi-t, lift it up with the tip of the scissors or a kocher.

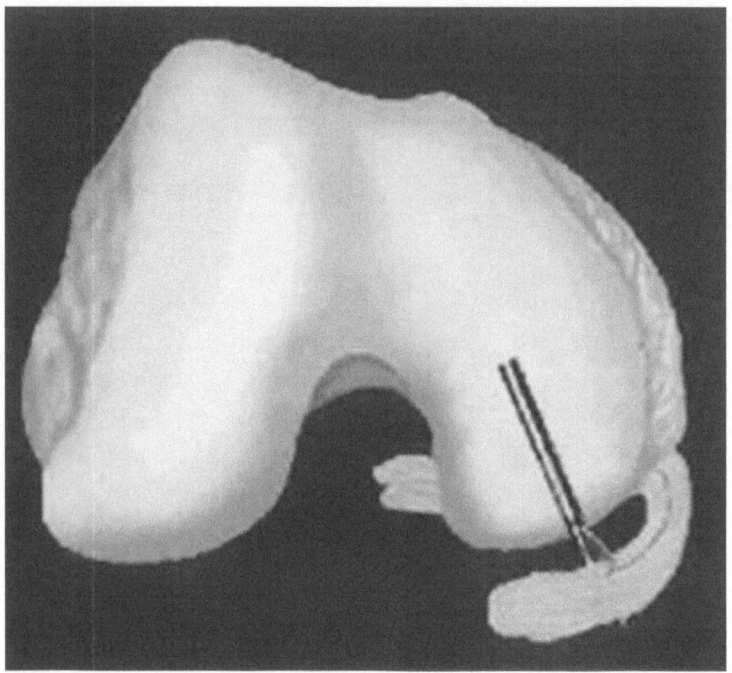

FIGURE 6.29. Cutting the anterior horn attachment of the meniscus.

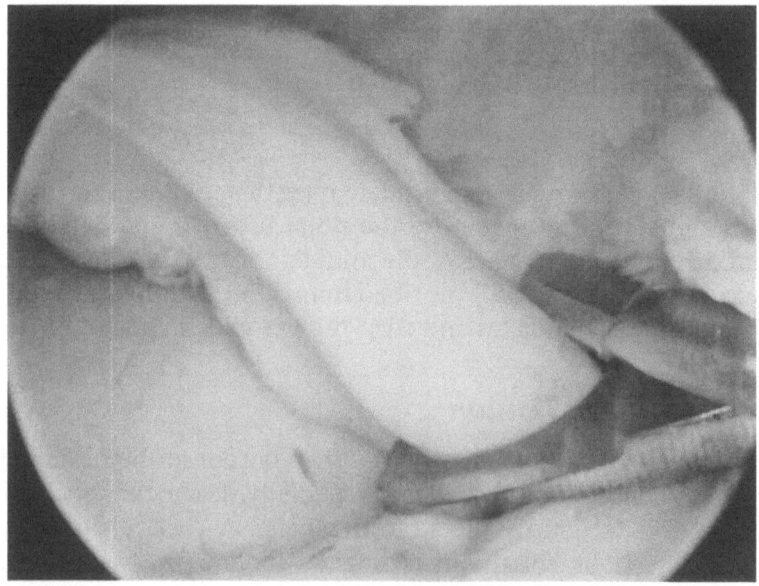

FIGURE 6.30. The arthroscopic view of cutting the anterior horn attachment.

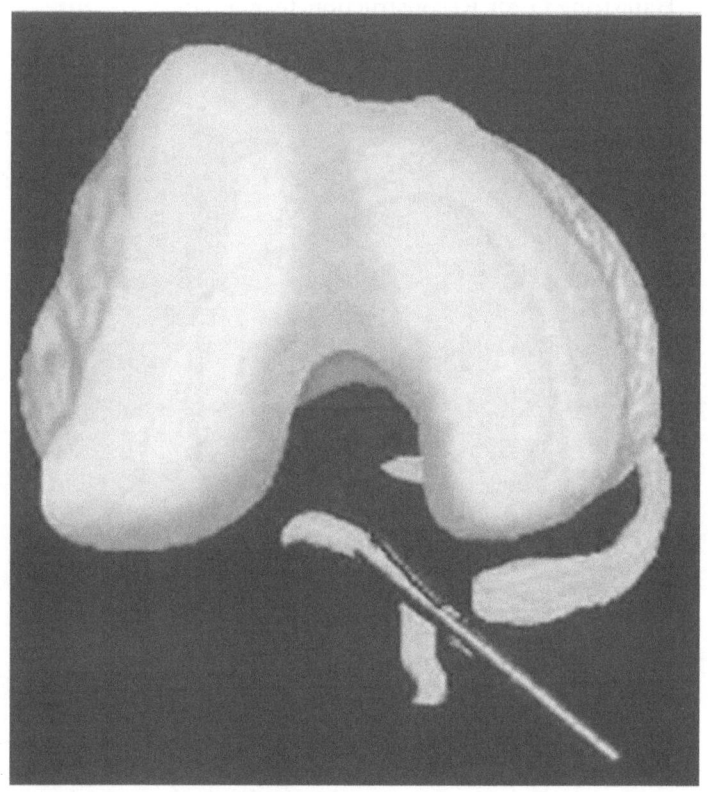

FIGURE 6.31. Removing the loose fragment with a grasper.

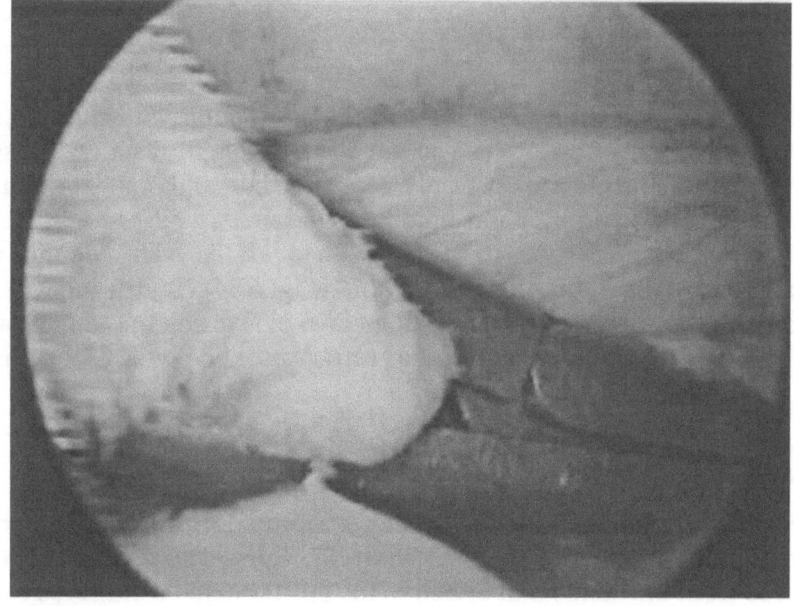

FIGURE 6.32. The removal of the loose fragment with the grasper.

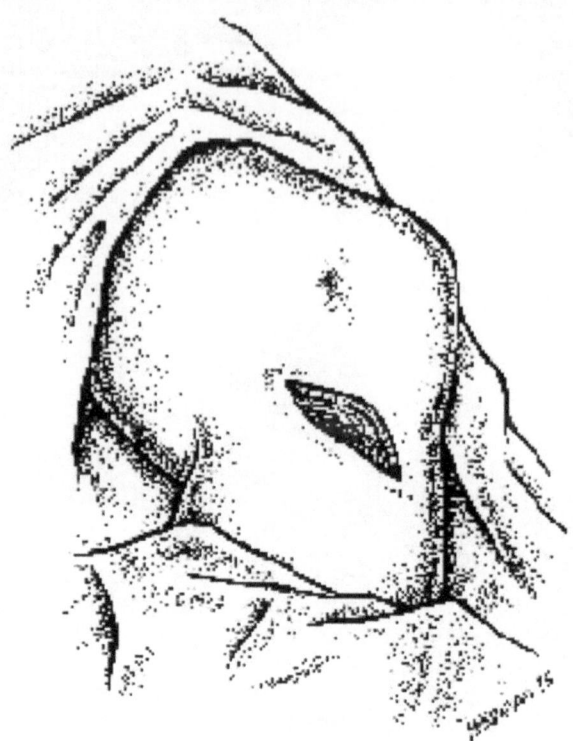

FIGURE 6.33. The skin incision for the hamstring tendon harvest.

Tendon Release

The first step is to free the distal end of the tendon with the scissors. The physician must make sure to get the full length distally. Grasp it with a kocher and traction it firmly. Many of the bands can be released with the traction and by blunt finger dissection.

The main band that goes to the medial head of the gastrocnemius will usually have to be cut with the scissors (Fig. 6.34). Pull firmly on the tendon and cut away from the tendon (to avoid cutting the tendon with the scissors). The tendon should not retract proximally if all the bands are cut.

Stripping of the Tendon

The tendon stripper is pushed up along the tendon to remove it from its muscular attachment (Fig. 6.35 and Fig. 6.36). The tendon must be cut free from the bands that attach to the gastrocnemius. If there is even

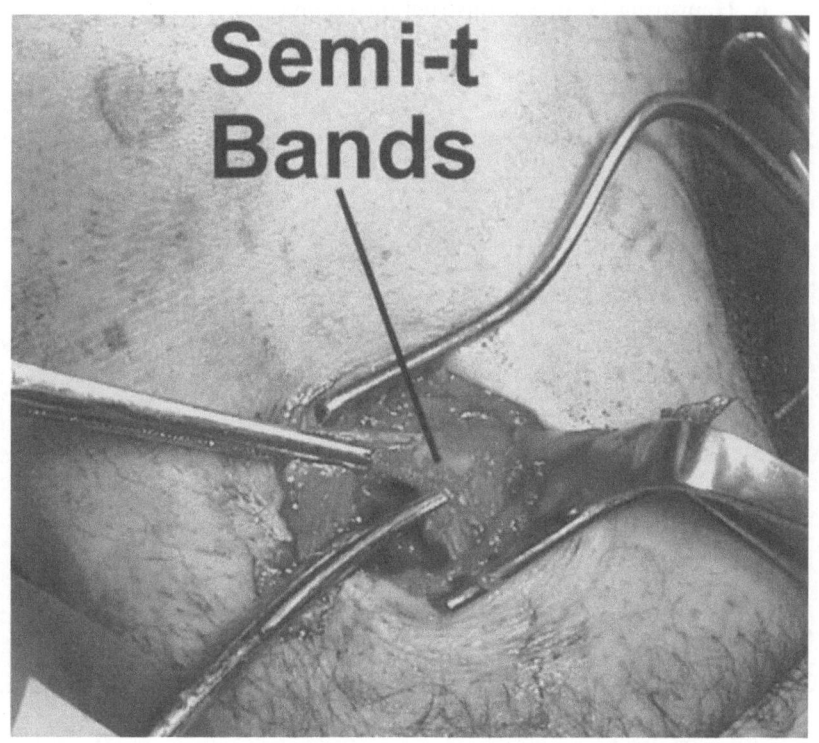

FIGURE 6.34. The release of the bands from the semi-t to the gastrocnemius.

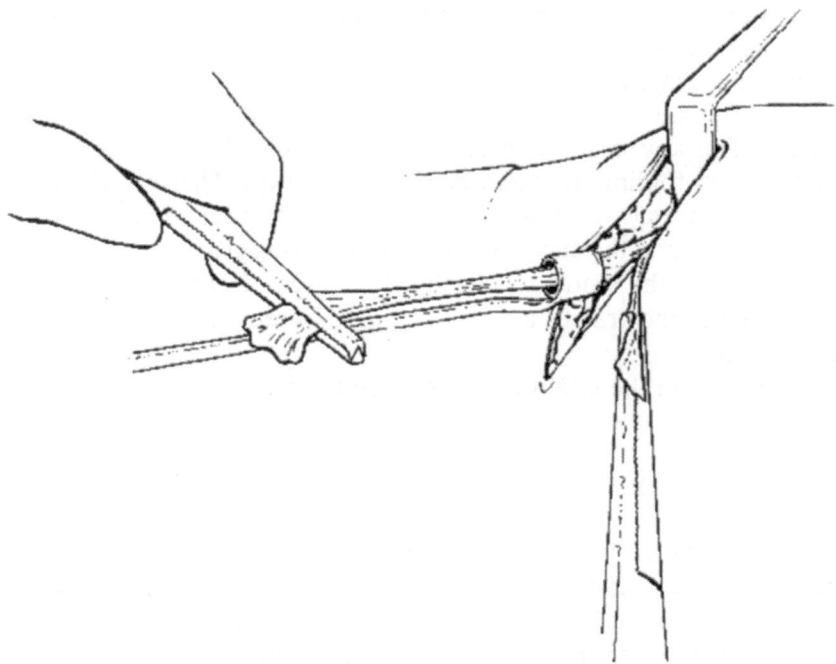

FIGURE 6.35. Stripping the tendons.

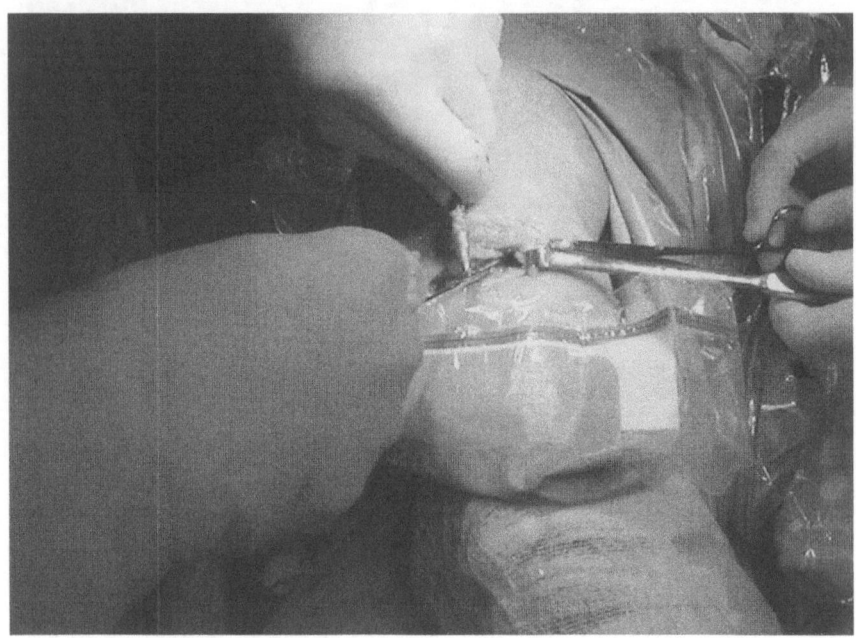

FIGURE 6.36. The stripping of the tendons with the closed-loop tendon stripper.

a small band, it causes the tendon to kink, and the stripper may cut it off short (Fig. 6.37).

The full length of the harvested tendon is usually about 30 cm (Fig. 6.38). The tendon stripper is pushed up the tendon using short strokes. The key is to keep tension on the distal end to prevent the tendon from folding over and being cut off short. There is often resistance at the muscle tendon junction, and the stripper should be rotated to slip it up along the surface of the muscle. This gives extra length. The total length of the tendon is usually 28 to 30 cm. If it is shorter, then the physician has the gracilis tendon. The gracilis tendon is harvested in the same fashion.

The video on the CD illustrates these procedures.

Preparation of the Graft

The graft is taken to the graft master on the back table. It is laid out, measured, and the muscle removed with the periosteal stripper. The ideal is to have four bundles of graft, 10 cm in length. The graft is folded over and leader sutures are placed in each end. The two tendons are

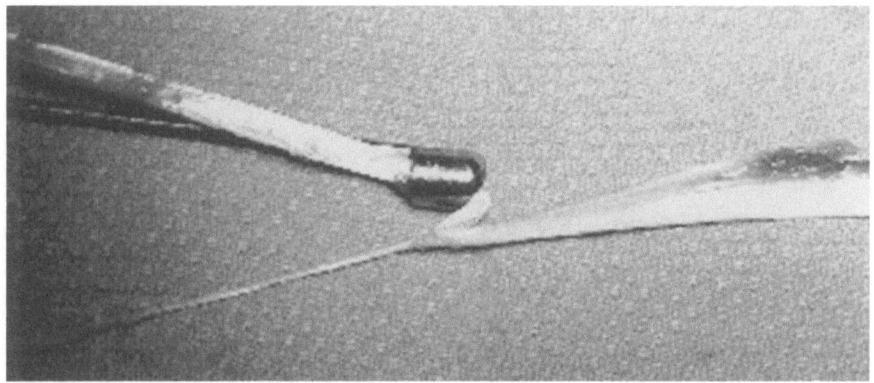

FIGURE 6.37. A small band from the gastrocnemius may kink the tendon causing the tendon stripper to cut it off short when it is advanced.

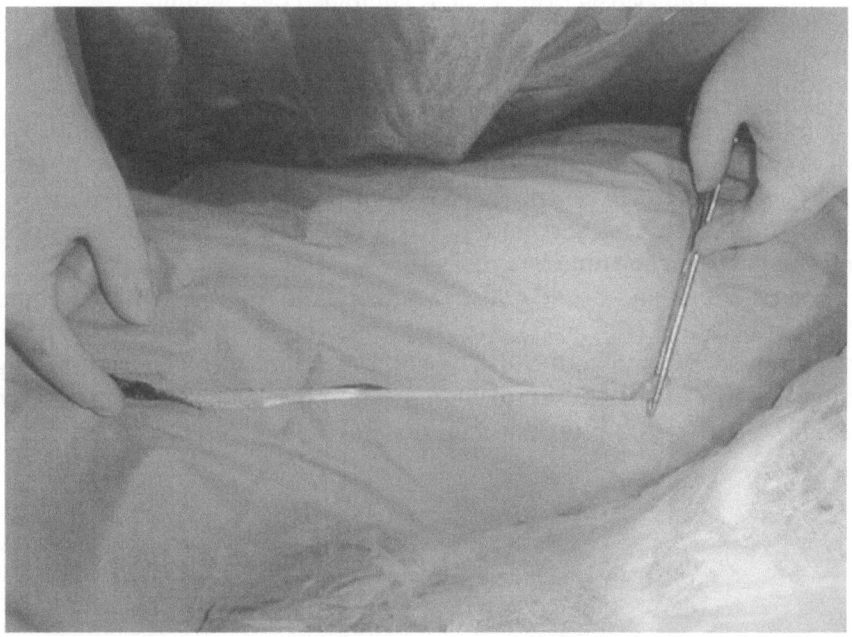

FIGURE 6.38. The completed harvest of the semitendinosus tendon.

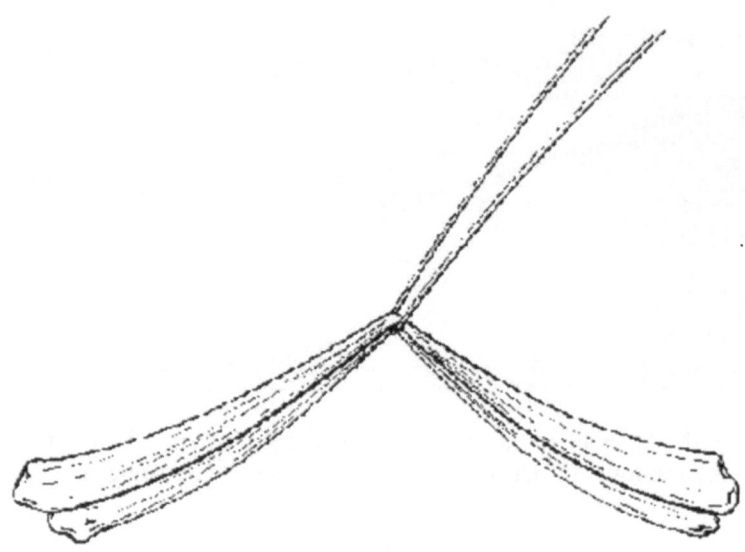

FIGURE 6.39. The tendons are folded over a suture.

folded over the number 5 Ti-Cron suture (Sherwood Medical, St. Louis, MO) (Fig. 6.39). The ends of the tendons are secured with two number 2 Ti-Cron suture (Fig. 6.40). The sutures are placed into the tendon over a length of 3 cm. This serves to act as a marker, when we are positioning the graft in the tunnels.

The proximal end of the graft is whipstitched together with a number 2 Ti-Cron suture (Fig. 6.41). This prevents the graft from wrapping up when the screw is introduced. The stitch is done over 3 cm to mark the length of graft in the femoral tunnel. The physician should mark 3 cm from the end with a blue skin marker pen.

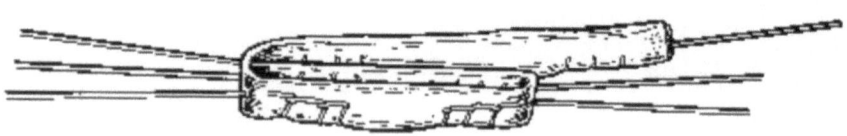

FIGURE 6.40. The distal ends of the tendon are whipstitched stitched together.

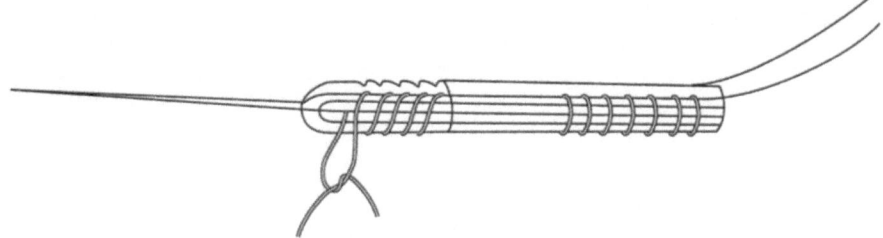

FIGURE 6.41. The proximal ends are also whipstitched together.

The final appearance of the prepared four-bundle, "Y"-hamstring graft is shown in Figure 6.42. The graft is then sized to the half size with a sizing cylinder (Fig. 6.43).

Endopearl Technique

The use of a secondary fixation on the femoral side is necessary in cases with reduced bone density. Fulkerson and Weiler have demonstrated that the use of a ball tied to the end of the tendon increases the ulti-

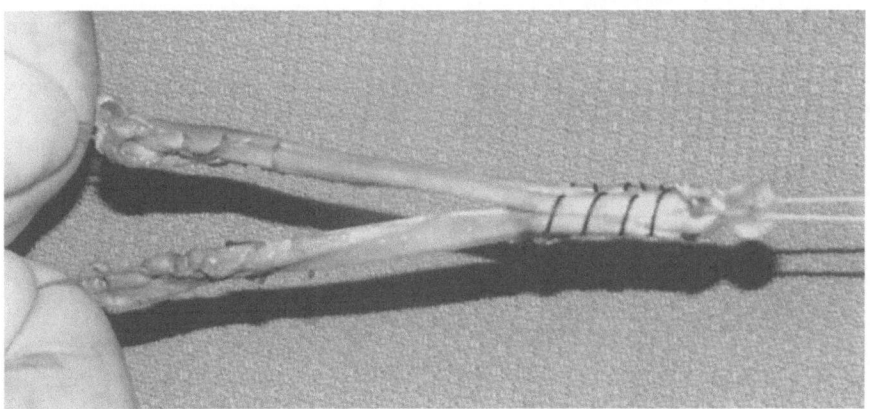

FIGURE 6.42. The final appearance of the graft.

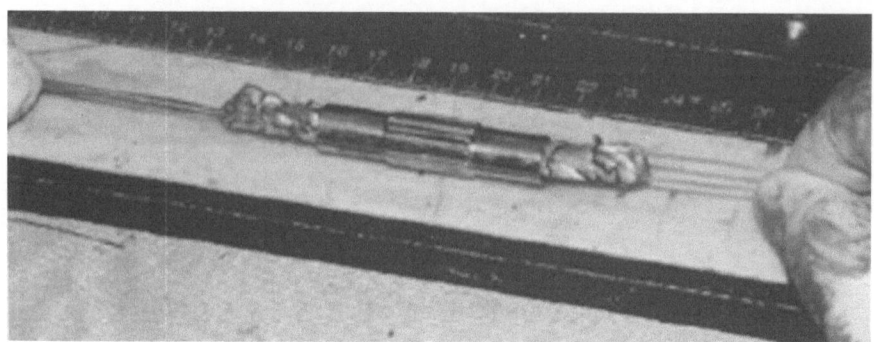

FIGURE 6.43. The graft is sized to the half centimeter.

mate load to failure, as well as significantly improving the slippage of the graft under the screw with cyclic loading.

The Endopearl is sutured to the proximal looped end of the semi-tendinosus and gracilis (Fig. 6.44). The proximal end of the graft is sutured together with number 2 Ti-Cron suture to prevent the graft from wrapping when the screw is inserted.

The tendon is marked just beyond the length of the screw as it abuts against the Endopearl (Fig. 6.45). This mark determines how far to pull the graft into the femoral tunnel. When the screw abuts against the Endopearl in the femoral tunnel, the pullout strength increases by 50%.

The video on the CD illustrates this procedure.

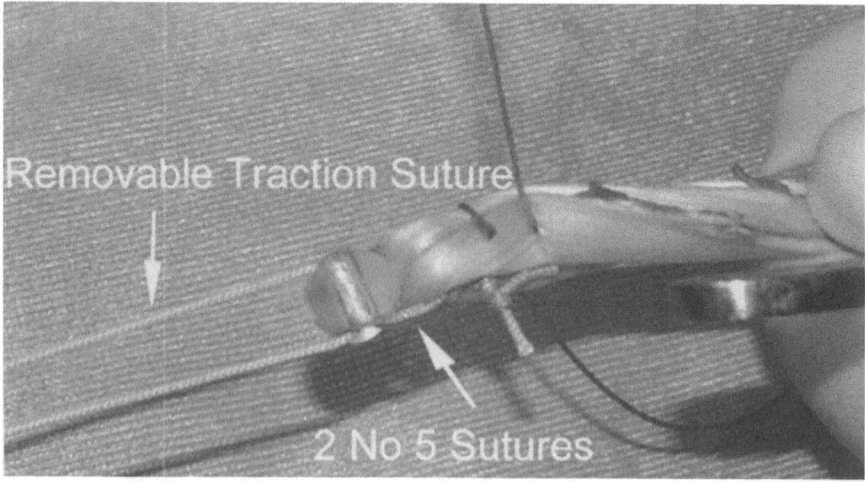

FIGURE 6.44. The Endopearl is sutured to the proximal end of the tendon.

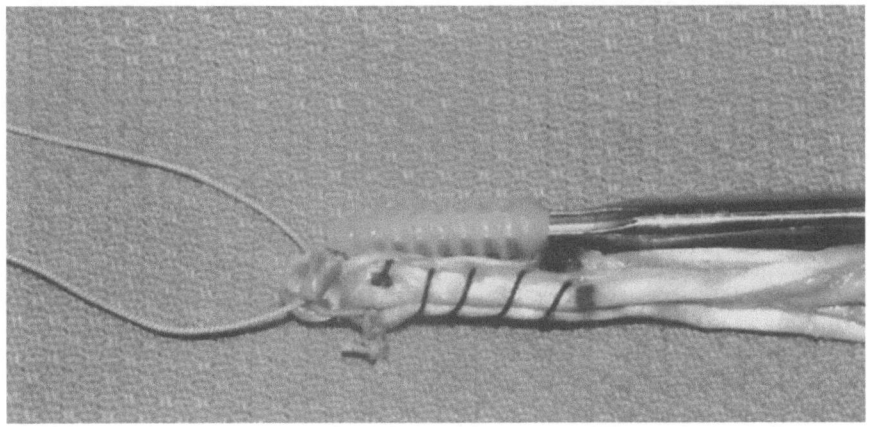

FIGURE 6.45. The Bioscrew and the Endopearl.

Graft Tensioning

This four-bundle graft will be four times the strength of a single strand of semi-t, as long as all bundles are tensioned (Fig. 6.46). The graft is incorporated into the bone tunnel by tendon ingrowth with Sharpey's fibers. This will take about 10 to 12 weeks to heal. This graft will have at least 3 cm of graft in each tunnel. The depth of graft in the tunnel can be determined by the 3 cm of suture marker at each end.

Notchplasty and ACL Stump Debridement

The ACL stump is removed with a combination of the shaver and the electrocautery. In most cases no bone is removed, only the soft tissue from the wall of the notch. There is still considerable controversy over the extent of the notchplasty. Some surgeons do a notchplasty in only 10% of their cases. Others always do one. The author thinks that the answer lies somewhere in between. Each physician should do what needs to be done to accommodate an 8 to 10 mm graft. In cases with a very narrow A-frame notch, this will mean more extensive use of the burr to remove enough bone to visualize the back of the notch (Fig. 6.47 and Fig. 6.48). Measure the size of the notch with an instrument, such as a pituitary rongeur that opens to 10 mm. Make the notch large enough to accept this 10-mm instrument. The emphasis should be on the roof and the anterolateral corner. Change the A-shape at the top of the notch to a U-shape.

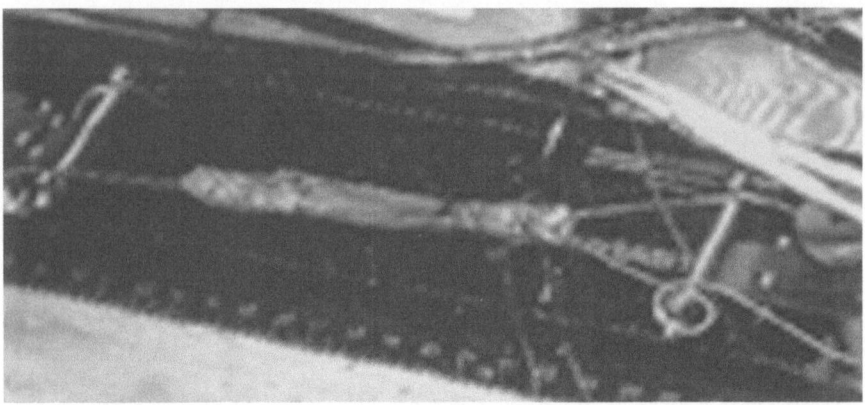

FIGURE 6.46. The tensioning of the graft on the graft preparation table.

It is important to remove the soft tissue to visualize the back of the notch. Use a large curette to lift the soft tissue off and then a 5.5-mm Gater (Linvatec, Largo, FL) resector to clean the notch (Fig. 6.49). The critical area to see is the fringe of capsule at the back. The residents ridge does not have this fringe, so the physician should easily identify the correct area. Put the pump pressure up at this stage to distend the

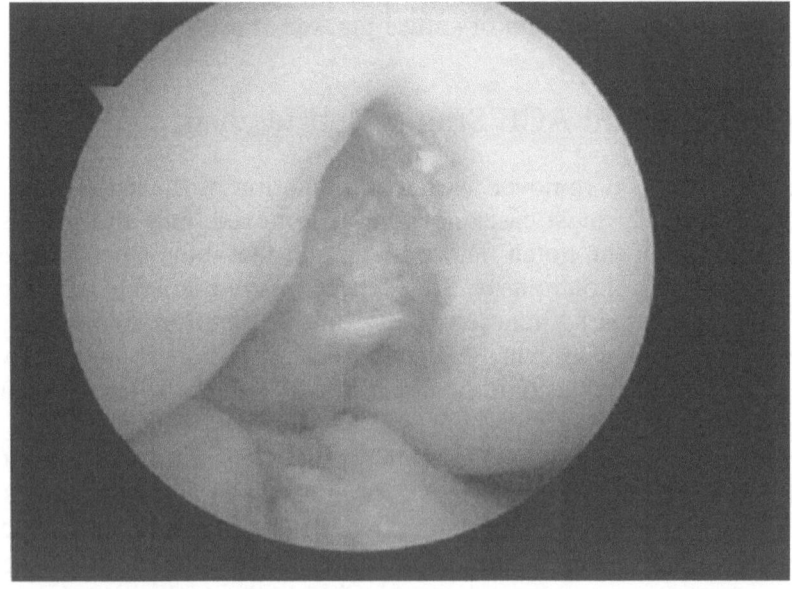

FIGURE 6.47. A stenotic A-frame notch.

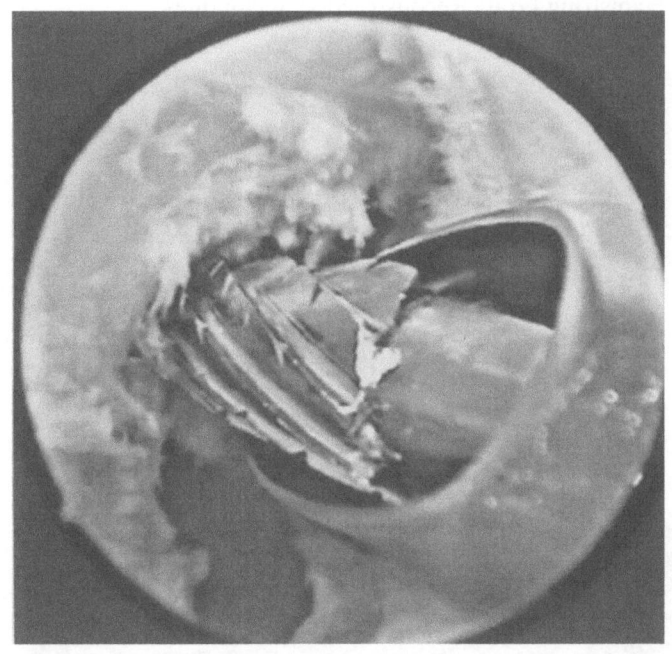

FIGURE 6.48. The use of a burr to open up the stenotic notch.

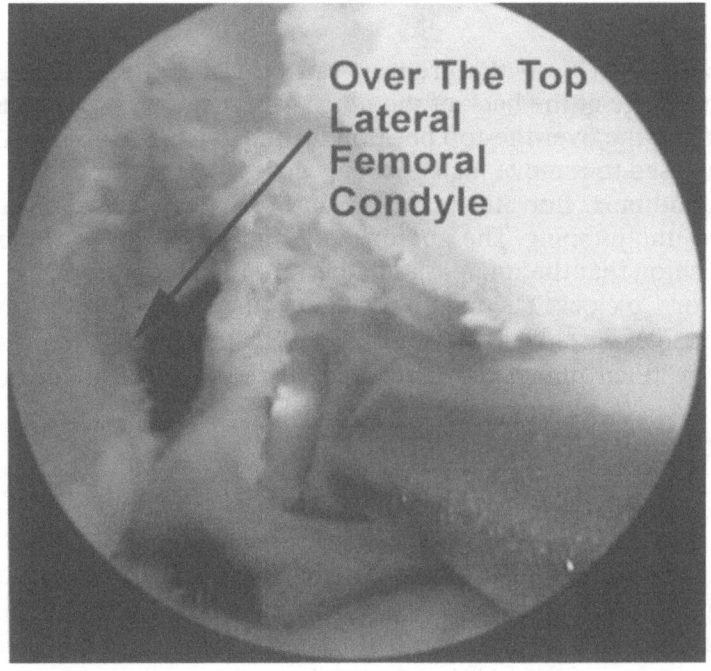

Over The Top
Lateral
Femoral
Condyle

FIGURE 6.49. The use of the curette to perform a soft tissue notchplasty.

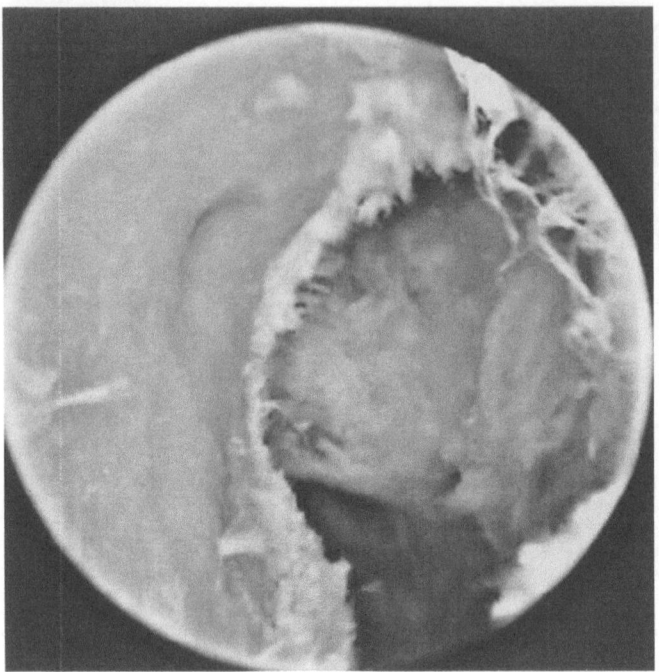

FIGURE 6.50. The completed notchplasty.

fat behind the PCL so the drop-off can be clearly seen. Figure 6.50 shows the fringe at the back of the notch, which the physician must see to determine the over-the-top position for the guide. A 6-mm oval burr should be used to remove the bone. This does not jump around as much as the round burr. Linvatec makes a southpaw for left knees that also eliminates the jumping. The author makes a small divot with the burr at the position that the tunnel should be, that is, 7 mm in from the drop-off at 11 or 1 o'clock. The major mistake would be not to clear enough soft tissue to expose the posterior aspect of the notch. This can result in drilling the tibial tunnel too anterior. The result is late failure of the graft.

Tibial Tunnel

Choosing the correct position for the tibial tunnel is crucial to the rest of the operation. The landmarks are external surface of the tibia, 4 cm from joint line, 2 cm medial to tibial tubercle; inside, 7 mm anterior to the leading edge of the PCL, in the midline.

The Linvatec tibial guide is set at 55° (Fig. 6.51). The guide is inserted through the anteromedial portal, by turning it upside down. The knee

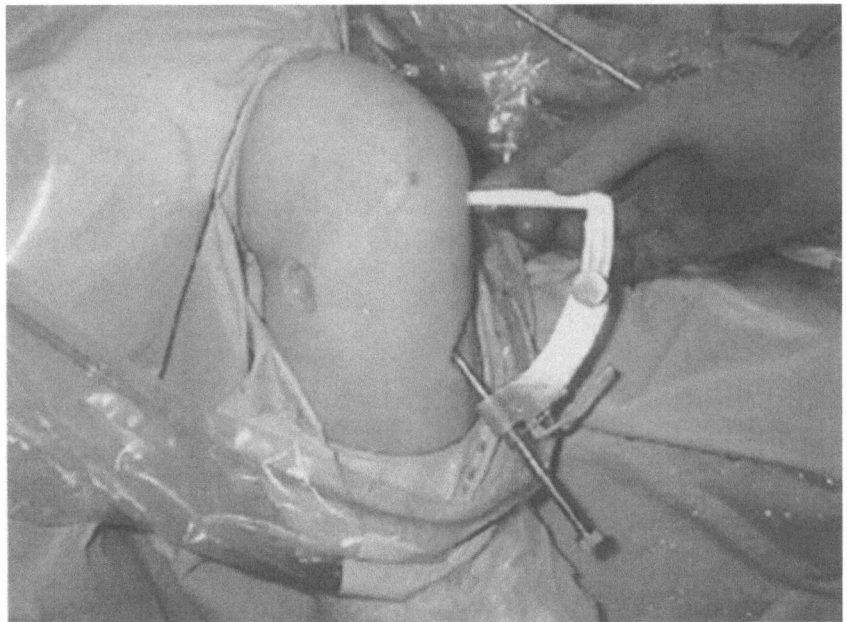

FIGURE 6.51. The Linvatec tibial guide.

is flexed to 90°. The distal point of the guide is positioned 2 cm medial to the tubercle and 4 cm from the joint line.

The tip, as shown in Figure 6.52 is placed in the midline between the spines and 7 mm anterior to the PCL. Drill a K-wire (Fig. 6.53) through the guide into the joint. When the wire hits the guide, loosen it and let the wire advance. It should just touch the leading edge of the PCL. Remove the guide. Ream over the K-wire with a 10-mm drill bit. Clean the interior tunnel site with the 5.5-mm Gater blade. If necessary, chamfer the posterior rim with the chamfering device on the drill. Clean the exterior tunnel site with the 5.5-mm Gater blade. This allows for easy passage of the graft. In the photo, this K-wire is in a good position. The wire is in the middle of the ACL stump, approximately 7 mm in front of the PCL, in the midline and just touching the edge of the PCL. The video on the CD demonstrates the tunnel procedure.

Femoral Tunnel

To drill the femoral tunnel, the Bullseye (Linvatec, Largo, FL) femoral aiming guide is placed through the tibial tunnel. This means that the tibial tunnel must be in the correct position and at the correct angle or it will be impossible to place the femoral tunnel correctly. The tunnels

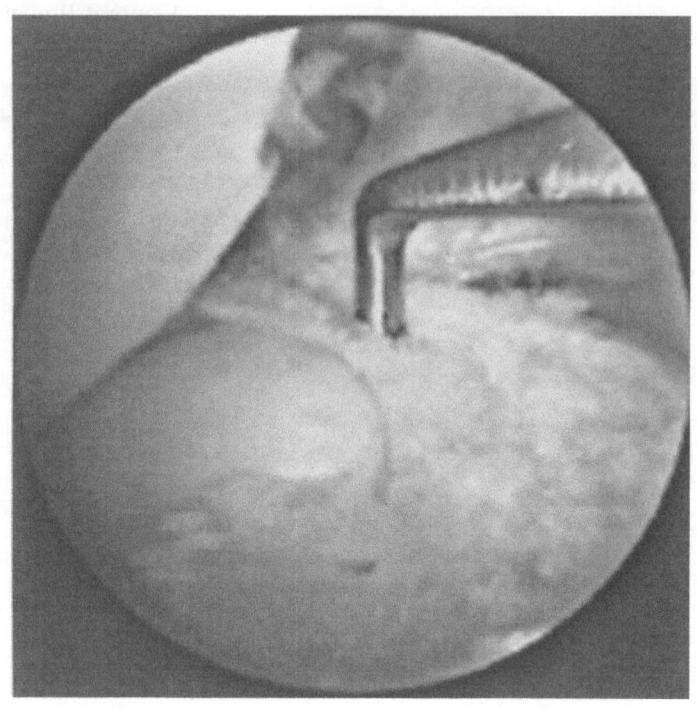

FIGURE 6.52. The tip placement of the tibial guide.

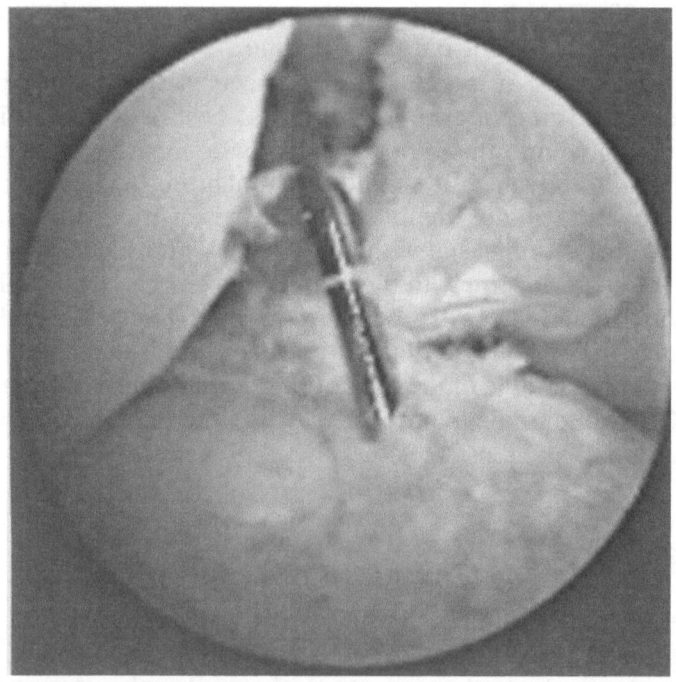

FIGURE 6.53. The ideal position for the tibial guide wire.

are drilled according to the graft measurement, that is, 7 or 8mm. The physician should not leave the graft soaking in saline, as it may swell and make passing difficult. The graft should simply be wrapped in a surgical sponge.

The femoral tunnel is drilled through the tibial tunnel with the use of the femoral aiming guide (Fig. 6.54). The Bullseye guide is inserted through the tibial tunnel, the flare of the guide placed over the top of the femoral condyle, and the guide aimed at the 11 or 1 o'clock position (Fig. 6.55). A long, guide-passing wire is drilled into the femur and retrieved through the anterolateral thigh. The surgeon should avoid placing the femoral tunnel in a vertical position. Howell has shown that the vertical graft provides a-p stability, but not rotational stability at 30° of knee flexion. The oblique position of the graft is preferable to the vertical graft position.

The guide wire (Linvatec, Largo, FL) is overdrilled with the same size C-reamer as used in the tibial tunnel. It is important to make a footprint on the condyle by drilling only half of the head of the drill bit into the bone. The drill bit is retracted and the footprint examined to determine if it is in the correct position (Fig. 6.56 and Fig. 6.57). The video on the CD illustrates this procedure.

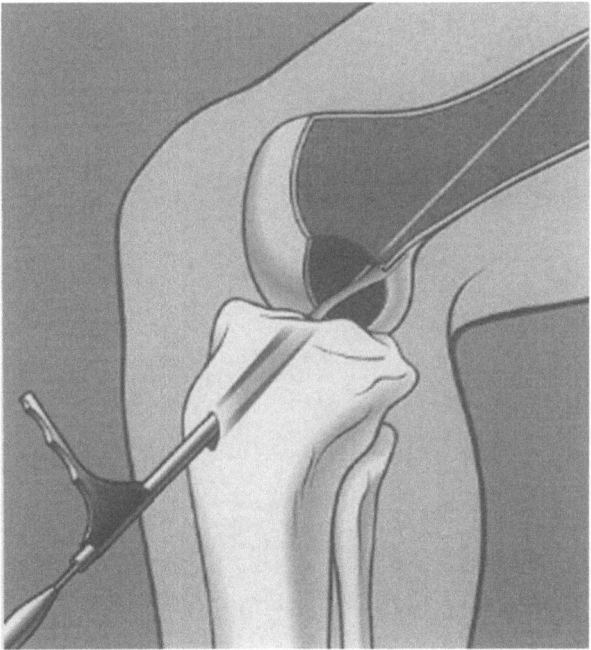

FIGURE 6.54. The transtibial Bullseye femoral aiming guide.

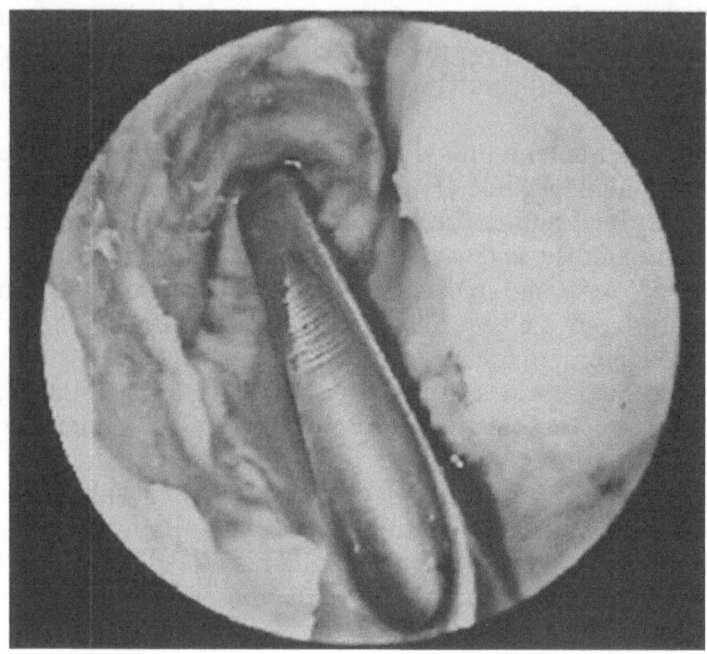

FIGURE 6.55. The position of the femoral aiming guide.

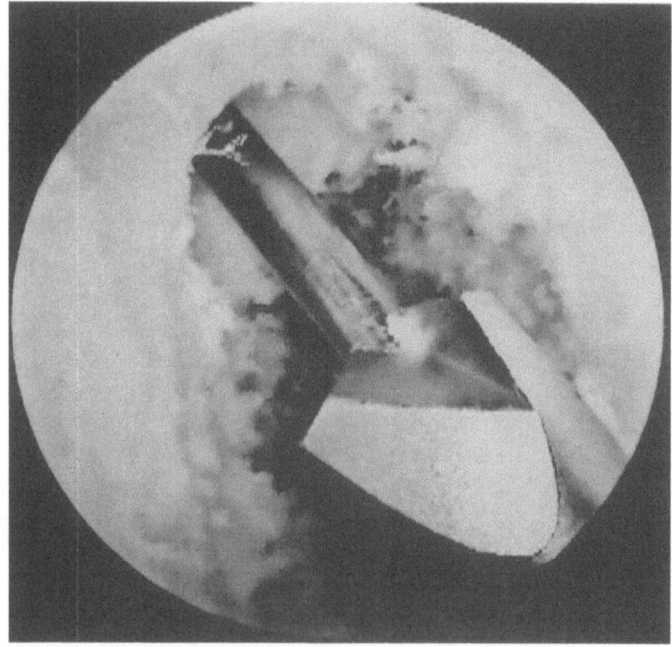

FIGURE 6.56. The footprint made by the drill bit.

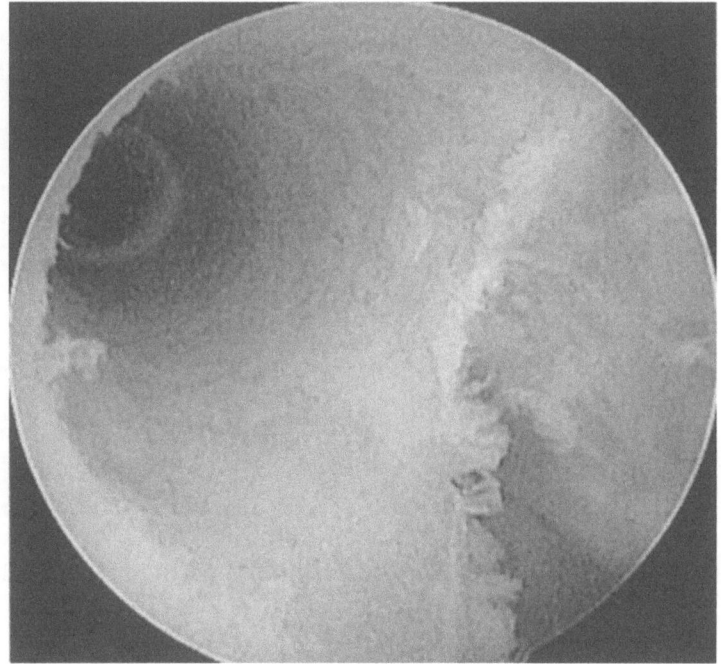

FIGURE 6.57. This demonstrates the ideal posterior wall of 1–2 mm.

Tunnel Dilation

Tunnel dilation is a method to compact the tunnel wall to improve the pullout strength of the interference screw. In the middle-aged patient, the tunnels should be dilated 2 sizes to improve the fixation strength. For example, if the graft is 8mm, drill a 6-mm tunnel and dilate 2 sizes. Drilling a small tunnel in both the tibia and femur and inserting the graft passing wire through both tunnels facilitates the dilation procedure. The tunnels are dilated up to the size of the composite graft. The tibial end is often a half size larger because of the suturing. With the graft passing wire inserted, both tunnels can be quickly dilated with a single pass of the dilators (Fig. 6.58).

Tunnel Notching

The edge of the tunnel must be notched to start the BioScrew (Linvatec, Largo, FL) (Fig. 6.59). This will allow the screw to start easily and avoid breaking the screw. The Notcher (Linvatec, Largo, FL) is inserted through the tibial tunnel to notch the femoral tunnel.

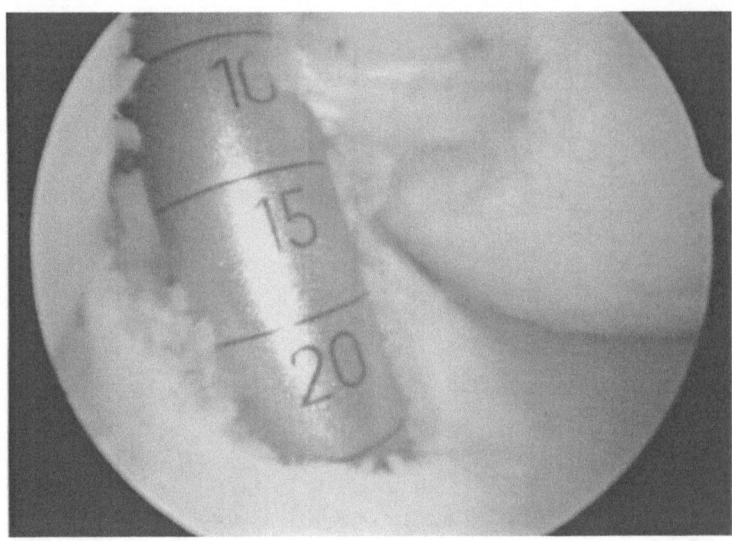

FIGURE 6.58. The use of metal dilators to compact the tunnel walls.

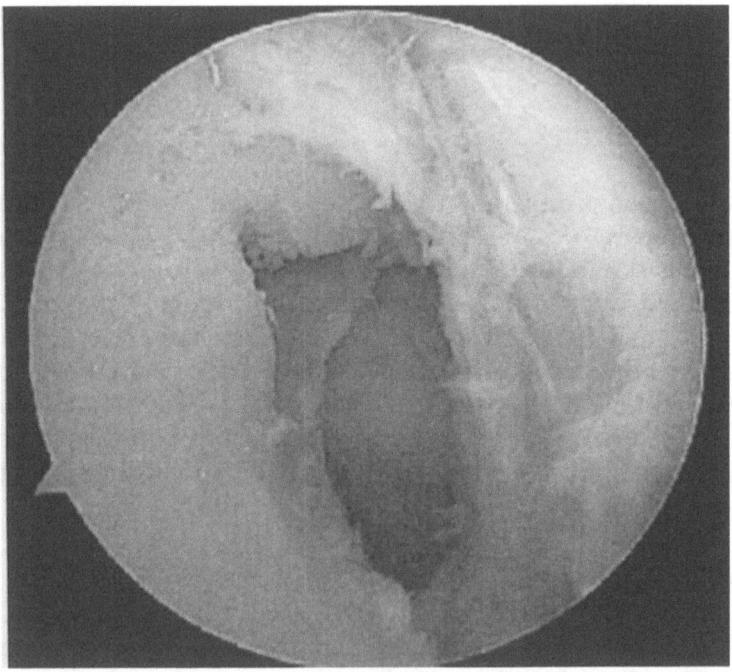

FIGURE 6.59. This demonstrates the notch in the edge of the tunnel to start the screw.

Graft Passage

The four-bundle semi-t and gracilis graft is attached to the looped end of the graft passing guide wire and the number 5 Ti-Cron is drawn into the femoral tunnel. The graft is pulled into the tibial tunnel. The knee is hyperflexed, and the BioScrew guide wire is introduced through the low anteromedial portal and into the notch in the femoral tunnel. The guide wire should lie on top of the graft, not pushed into the graft. The wire is shoehorned on top of the graft as it is pulled into the tunnel.

Figure 6.60 shows the leader suture pulling the Endopearl and the graft through the notch. The graft is drawn up to the edge of the femoral tunnel, and the flexible BioScrew guide wire is laid on top of the graft at the notched region of the tunnel (Fig. 6.61). The graft and the flexible guide wire are pulled into the femoral tunnel. The graft is pulled up to the blue mark on the graft (30 mm). If there is graft hanging out the tibial tunnel, it is pulled further into the femoral tunnel. The graft should be inside the tibial tunnel in case the fixation needs to be augmented with a periosteal button.

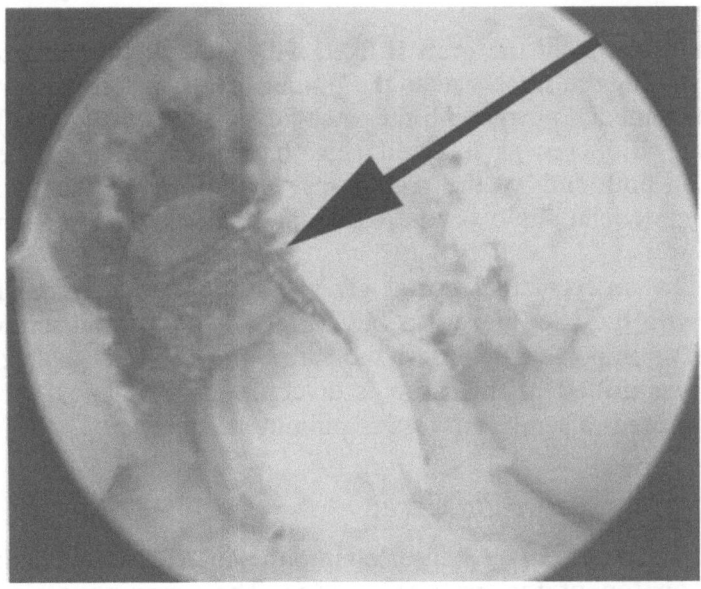

FIGURE 6.60. The Endopearl and hamstring graft passage.

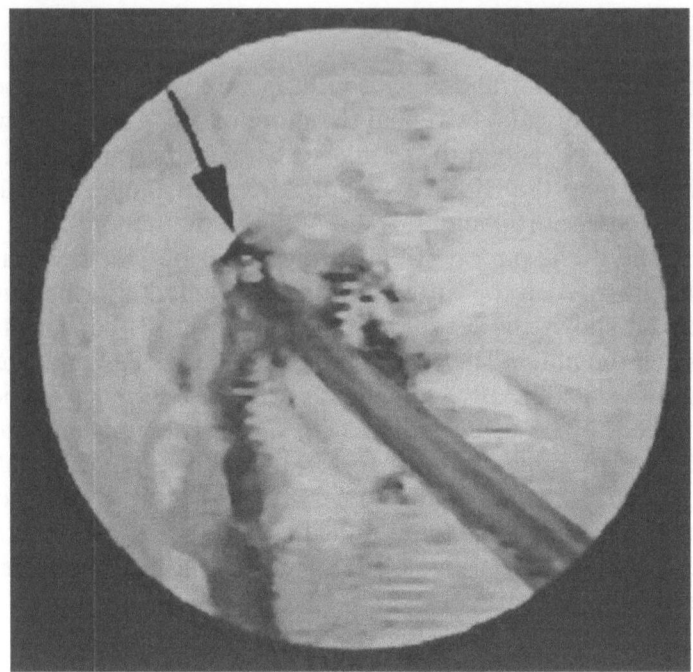

FIGURE 6.61. The guide wire inserted into the notch of the tunnel.

Graft Fixation

The femoral end of the graft is fixed with the appropriate sized Bio-Screw, usually the same size as the tunnel. This is inserted through the low anteromedial portal with the knee flexed at 110° (Fig. 6.62).

As the BioScrew is inserted (Fig. 6.63), tension must be maintained on both ends of the graft to prevent the screw from wrapping up the graft. The video on the CD demonstrates the insertion of the BioScrew.

The low anteromedial portal gives a straight shot at the femoral tunnel with the knee flexed to 110° (Fig. 6.64). To avoid screw divergence, it is important to insert the screw in the same angle that the tunnel was drilled. If the screw is divergent more than 15° from the tunnel, there is a significant loss of pullout strength.

Insertion of the Tibial Screw

The BioScrew guide wire is inserted into the anterior aspect of the tibial tunnel, on top of the graft (Fig. 6.65). The screw (one size larger than the tunnel) is inserted up the tibial tunnel to the internal aperture of the tunnel. Maintain tension on the leader sutures out the tibial

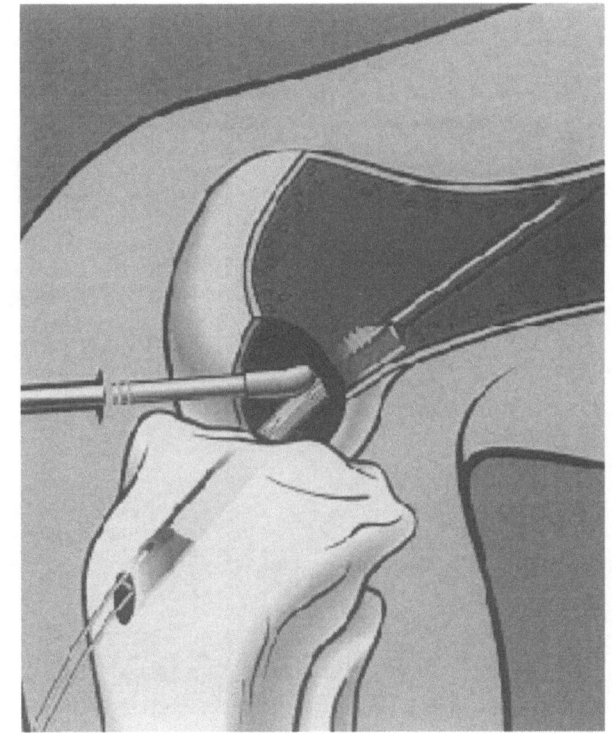

FIGURE 6.62. The insertion of the BioScrew through the anteromedial portal.

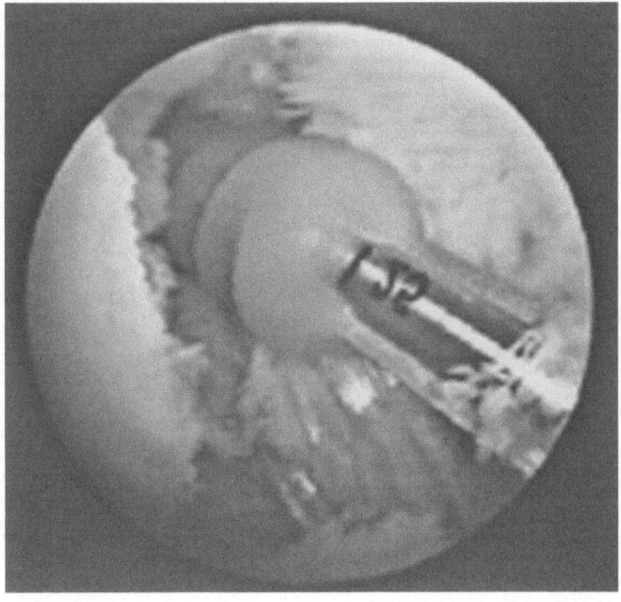

FIGURE 6.63. The insertion of the BioScrew into the femoral tunnel.

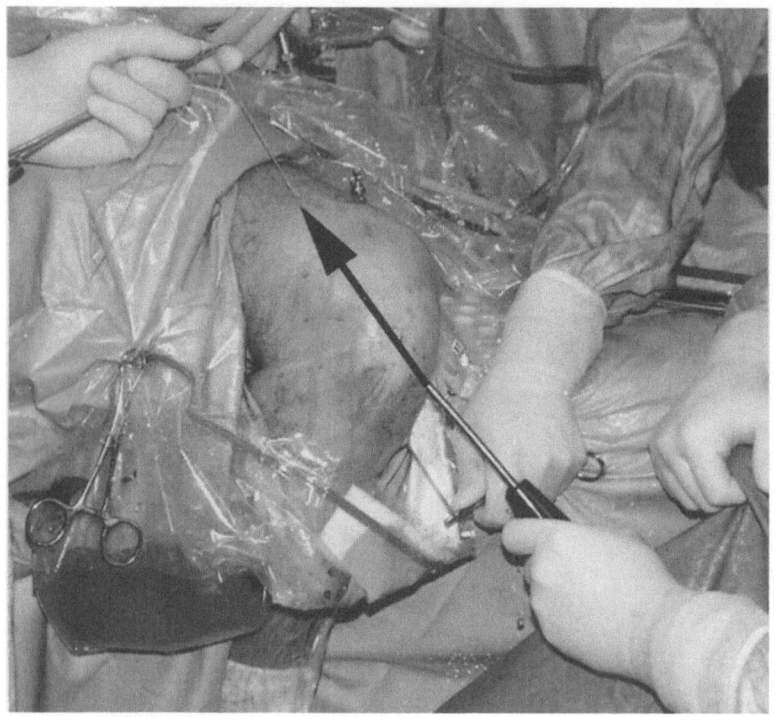

FIGURE 6.64. The low anteromedial portal gives a straight shot at the femoral tunnel with the knee flexed to 110°.

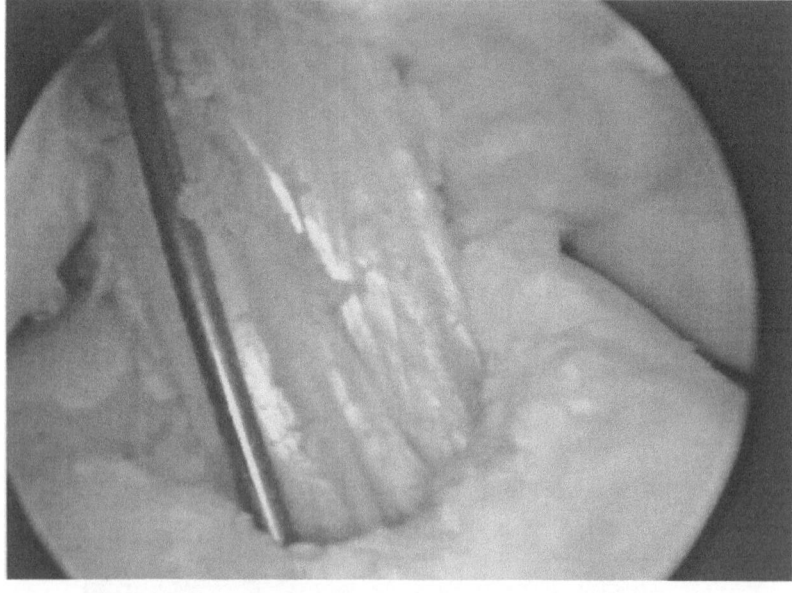

FIGURE 6.65. The tibial BioScrew guide wire inserted anterior to the graft.

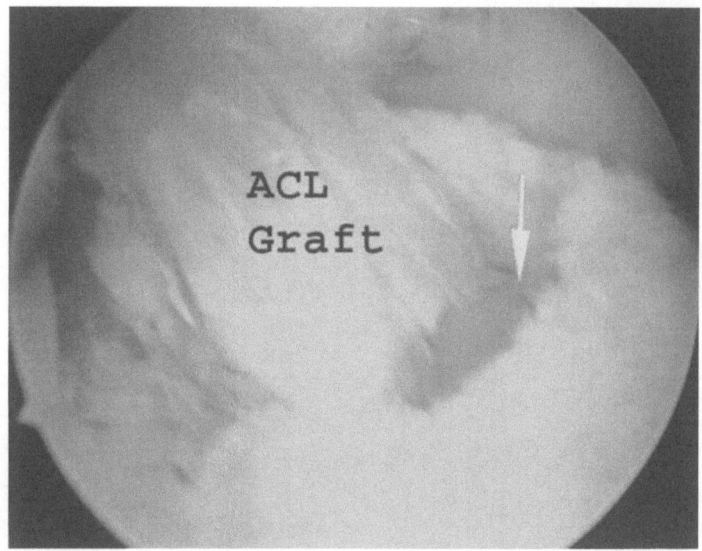

FIGURE 6.66. The screw tip can just be visualized at the internal tibial tunnel opening.

tunnel. This prevents pushing the graft up in front of the screw, thereby resulting in a loose graft. The knee flexion angle should be 15° when the graft is tensioned and the screw inserted. The tibial screw compresses the graft against the tunnel wall, but does not push the graft up the tunnel (Fig. 6.66 and Fig. 6.67). The leader sutures from the ends of the tendons are tied over a periosteal button to augment the tibial screw fixation (Fig. 6.68).

Graft Inspection: Look and Hook

The graft is inspected as the knee is moved through a range of motion, looking for anterior impingement and lateral wall abrasion (Fig. 6.69). The hook is used to assess tension in the graft. A manual Lachman test is done watching the motion of the tibial spine.

KT-S Measurements

Before the sutures are cut, the KT-S is used to pull a manual maximum number. This is compared to the normal side. If the other side is not normal, then 5 to 7 is taken as normal. Generally the manual maximum a-p translation will be equal or 1 to 2mm less than the opposite side (Fig. 6.70). Approximately 10% of the time, the difference is greater

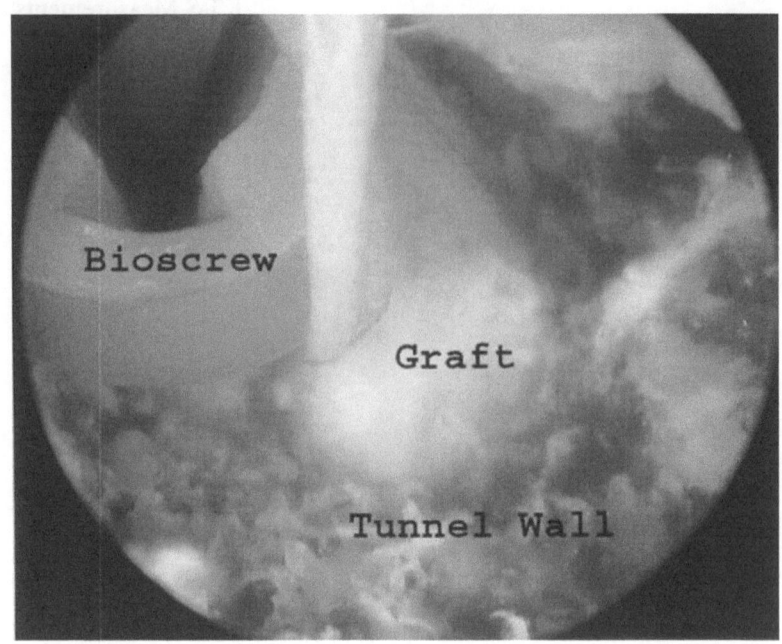

FIGURE 6.67. The tunneloscopy of the tibial screw.

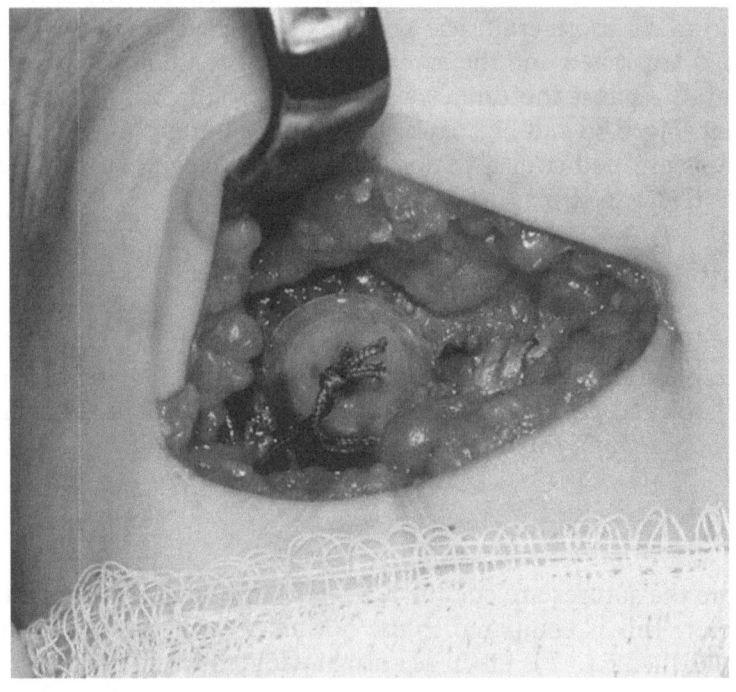

FIGURE 6.68. The secondary tibial fixation with a button.

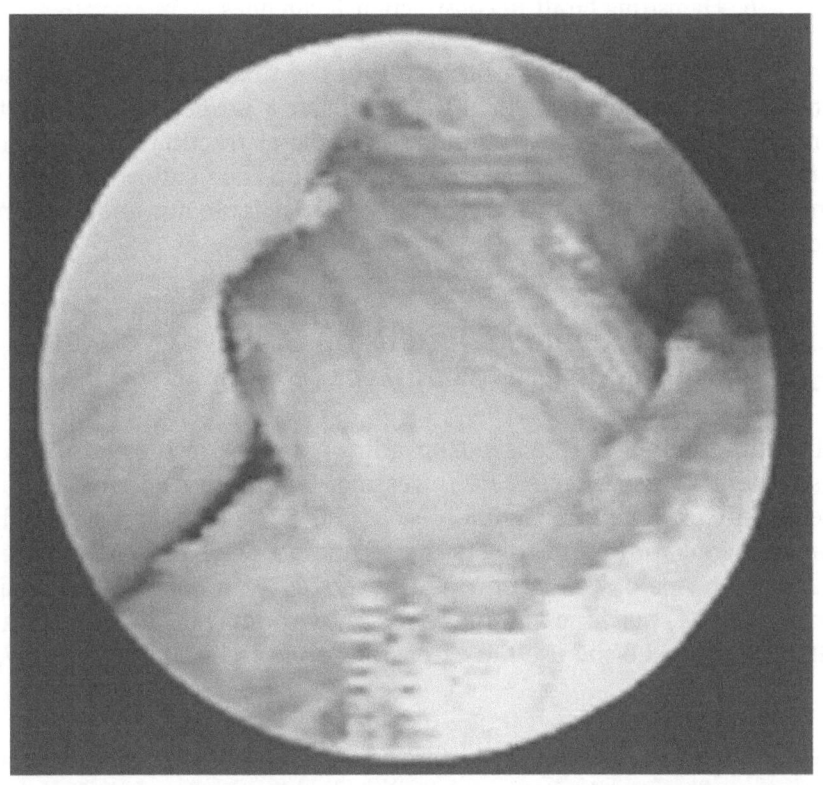

FIGURE 6.69. The completed four-bundle hamstring graft.

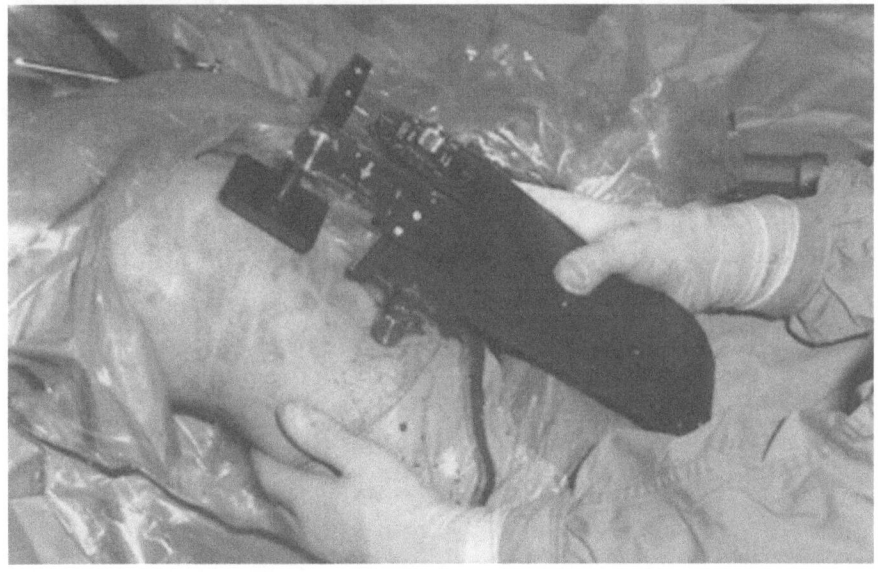

FIGURE 6.70. The final measurement of the a-p translation with the KT-S.

than 3mm. The tensioning of the graft at the tibial end is then revised. One common problem is when the tibial screw pushes the graft up the tunnel. The surgeon must maintain firm distal traction on the leader sutures to prevent the screw from grafting up. The sutures are cut off when the surgeon is satisfied that the knee is stable and the fixation is secure.

Postoperative Regimen: Extension Splint, Cryo-Cuff, and Continuous Passive Motion Machine

After the wounds are closed, the author applies a Tegaderm (Sklar Instruments, West Chester, PA) dressing, a compressive stocking and the Cryo-Cuff (Aircast, Summit, NJ) (Fig. 6.71). This is a sleeve that contains cool water and lowers the temperature of the knee, thereby reducing the pain. The patient is transferred to a continuous passive motion (CPM) machine and to the recovery room (Fig. 6.72). When the patient gets up, he/she use the extension splint and crutches (Fig. 6.73).

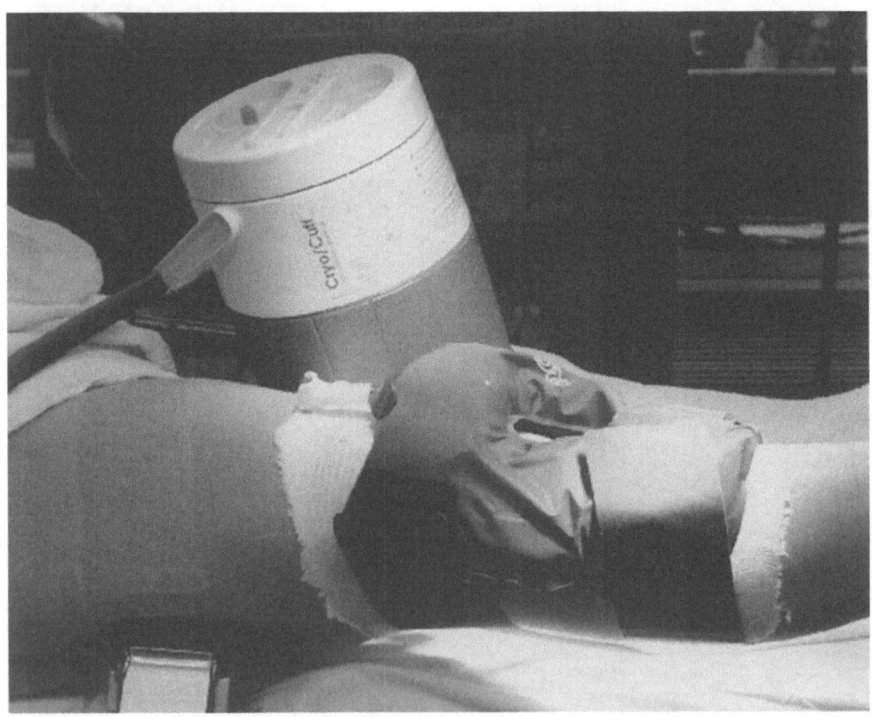

FIGURE 6.71. The Cryo-Cuff is applied to the knee in the operating room.

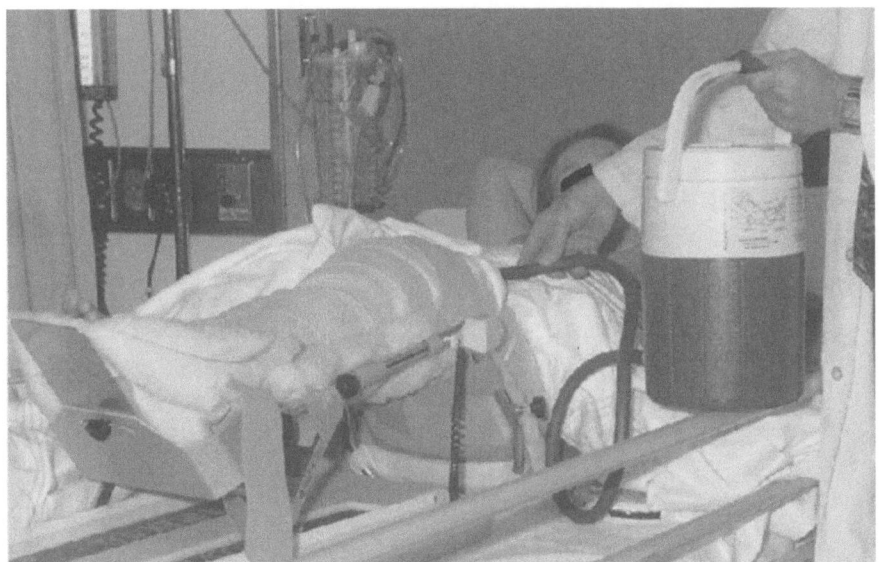

FIGURE 6.72. The CPM and Cryo-Cuff used immediately postoperatively.

The patient goes home several hours postoperatively with the CPM, the Cryo-Cuff, the extension splint, and crutches. Oral pain medication is 25 mg of Vioxx od, and Tylenol # 3 at 1 or 2 q.4.h. prn. The patient also receives 1 more intravenous dose of antibiotic. The patient returns for a checkup in four to five days. The Tegaderm dressing is removed, and the Cryo-Cuff applied directly to the skin. The wounds are cleansed for the next few days with 3% hydrogen peroxide.

Physiotherapy starts within four to five days. The author has a protocol that can be mailed to remote physiotherapy locations to ensure that the early extension routine is started. Routine checkups are monthly until the patient has fully recovered. The physician should try to get KT-1000 measurements at 6 weeks and at 3, 6, and 12 months. If there is any loss of extension, this is addressed early by vigorous aggressive rehabilitation. If there is still loss at three months, surgical debridement is suggested.

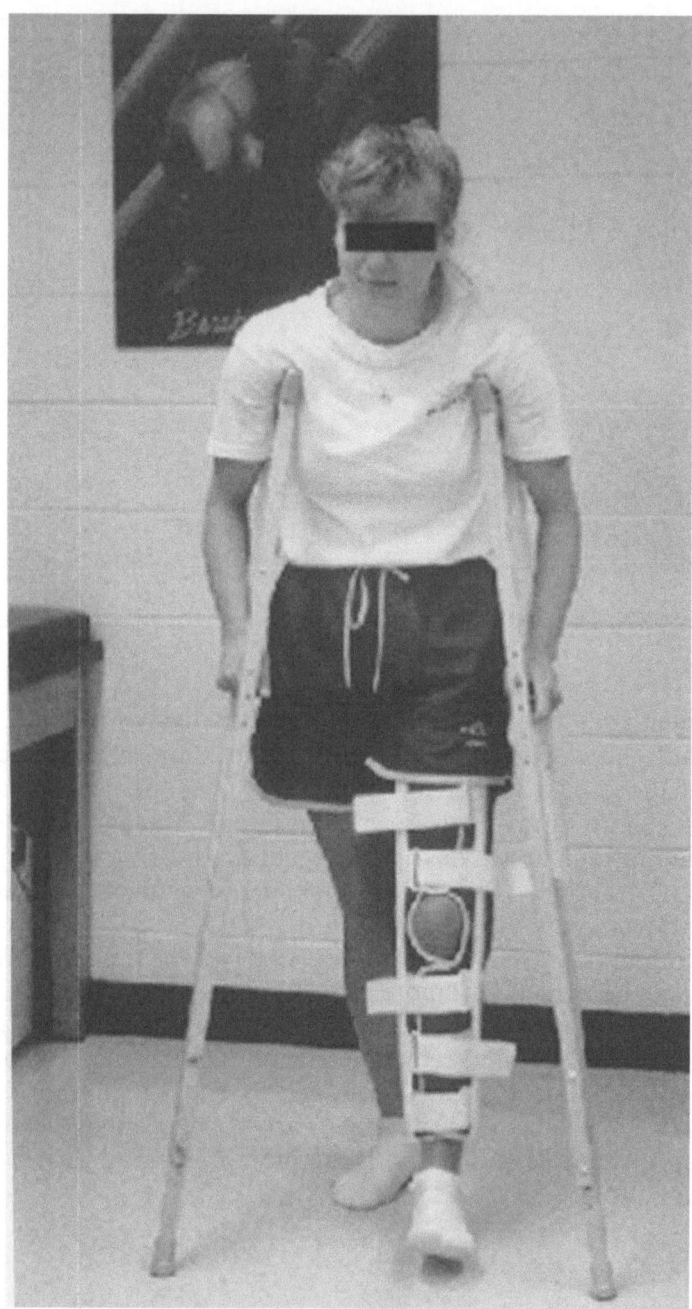

Figure 6.73. Crutches and an extension splint are used for the first few days postoperative when ambulating.

7
Patellar Tendon Graft Technique

The steps of the patellar tendon graft ACL reconstruction are as follows:

Preoperative assessment.
Diagnostic/operative arthroscopy.
Graft harvest.
Graft preparation.
Notchplasty.
Tibial tunnel.
Femoral tunnel.
Graft passage.
Graft tensioning and fixation.
Graft inspection.
KT-S measurements.
Postoperative regimen.

Some of the prepration for the procedures described in this chapter is the same as for the procedures discussed in Chapter 6. They are repeated here for the sake of completeness.

EUA, KT-1000 Measurements, Joint Injection, and Femoral Nerve Block

First confirm which is the correct side. The physician's initials (Fig. 7.1) should be visible on the correct knee. The low profile leg holder is high on the thigh to allow the graft passing wire to penetrate the anterolateral thigh. The tourniquet is placed proximal under the leg holder.

Preemptive Pain Management

In a recently published paper, we documented the benefit of the preemptive use of the femoral nerve block, intravenous injections, and local knee injections. The anesthetist uses a peripheral nerve stimulator

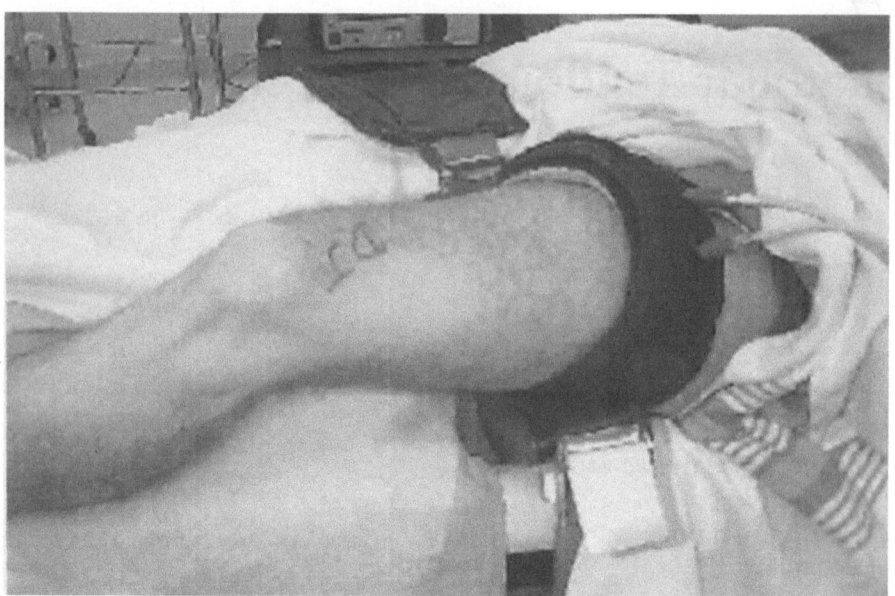

FIGURE 7.1. The setup for ACL reconstruction.

before the arthroscopy to block the femoral nerve (Fig. 6.4). The dosage is 20 cc of 0.25% bupivacaine with adrenaline. The knee joint and the incisions are injected with 20 cc of bupivacaine 0.25% with epinephrine and 2 mg of morphine. The patient has taken 50 mg of Vioxx orally one hour before, and the anesthetist gives 1 gm Ancef intravenously.

The physician is now ready to prepare and drape. Use a tourniquet inflated to 300 mm of mercury. The author uses a Linvatec (Largo, FL) fluid pump that works in coordination with the Apex driver system for the shaver and burrs to coordinate the flow level. A low profile leg holder is placed around the tourniquet. The knee is flexed over the side of the bed.

Diagnostic, Operative Arthroscopy

The diagnostic arthroscopy should be done before the graft harvest if there is any doubt about the diagnosis of partial versus complete ACL tear. This will confirm the presence of the ACL tear. The video on the CD illustrates this process, as well as the inside view of the "W," as discussed in Chapter 2.

The ACL must be carefully examined. The degree of tear must be assessed. The conventional wisdom is that a tear more than 50% should be reconstructed. But a partial tear, one of less than 50%, may have to be reconstructed with a patellar tendon. If the tear is minimal, with a negative pivot shift, this patient should be treated conservatively.

A complete diagnostic arthroscopy should be performed before any meniscal work is done. This ensures that the physician will not forget the lateral compartment if a lot of time is required to perform meniscal repair on the medial side. Assess the entire joint and plan the operative work. In young patients, every attempt should be made to repair the meniscus rather than resect it. The long-term results of reconstruction are more related to the state of the meniscus than to the stability.

A flap tear of the meniscus will cause pain, swelling, catching and giving way (Fig. 7.2). The flap is easily resected with a basket forceps and a motorized shaver. Figure 7.3 shows a bucket-handle tear of the medial meniscus that has displaced into the notch and is blocking exten-

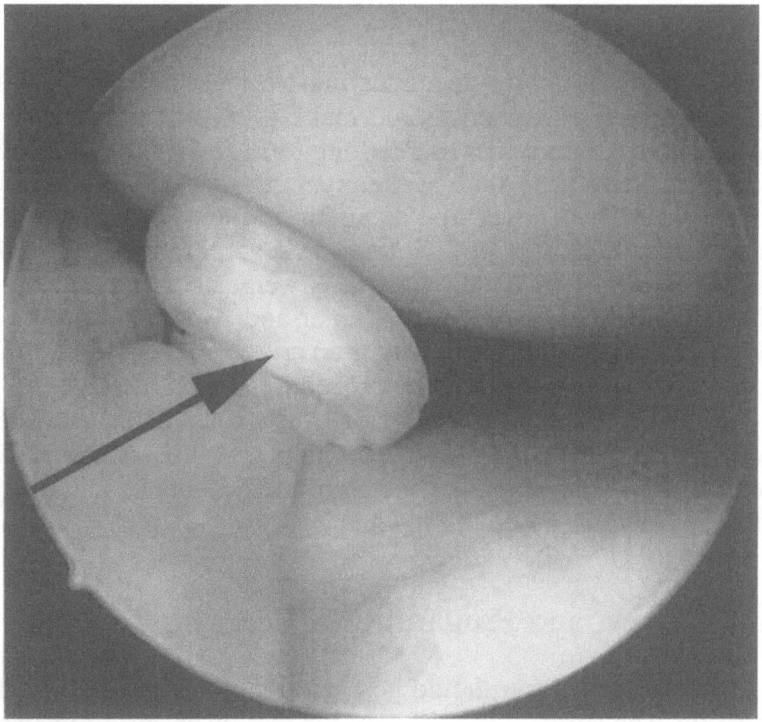

FIGURE 7.2. The flap tear (*arrow*) of the meniscus that produces mechanical symptoms.

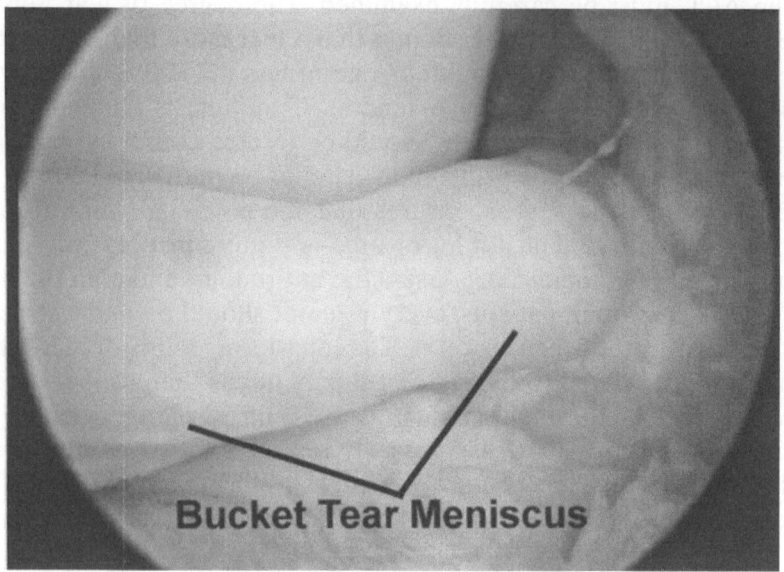

Bucket Tear Meniscus

FIGURE 7.3. The displaced bucket-handle tear of the meniscus.

sion. In this situation, the meniscus must be resected or repaired. In young patients, the surgeon should make every attempt to repair the meniscus rather than resect it. The long-term results of reconstruction are more related to the state of the meniscus than to the stability. The debate is whether to repair the meniscus and do the ACL reconstruction at the same sitting. This depends on several factors. If the limitation of extension is mild, the patient is weight bearing and the graft choice is hamstrings, the meniscus repair and ACL reconstruction can be done in one sitting. If the patient is on crutches with a significant lack of extension, for example 40°, the procedure should be staged to avoid postoperative stiffness. The meniscus repair is carried out, and when the patient has regained full range of motion, an ACL reconstruction is done. For the management of the associated meniscus pathology, see the hamstring graft, described in Chapter 6.

Graft Harvest and Preparation

The longitudinal incision should be 8 to 10 cm long and 1 cm medial to the tendon. The surgeon should plan for the lower end to incorporate the tibial tunnel. The incision can be as short as 5 cm if cosmetic appearance is important. The author has used two separate transverse incisions in the past, but prefers, in a teaching situation, to use the longitudinal incision. Studies have shown that the two transverse incisions do not injure the infrapatellar branch of the nerve, and the patients are able to kneel after the patellar tendon harvest.

A double-bladed knife cuts a 10-mm wide graft from the central third of the tendon (Fig. 7.4). The surgeon should mark the length of the bone plugs, patella: 2.5 cm, tibia: 3.5 cm.

A Hall (Linvatec, Largo, FL) microoscillating saw is used to cut the bone plugs (Fig. 7.5). The initial cut is vertical through the cortex for 4 to 5 mm. Then the saw is angled at 60° and cut to 8 mm in depth. A deep V-cut should be avoided, as it can lead to a stress riser and late fracture. A 1/16-in. drill bit is used to make two holes in each bone plug. The bone plugs are gently lifted out with a small 1-cm wide osteotome. The base of the bone plug should be flat. The graft is freed from the fat pad with scissors.

If the bone plug is cut too thin, or fractured, then the fixation will have to be augmented by tying the sutures over a screw post or a button. The video on the CD demonstrates the technique of patellar tendon harvest.

The transfer of the graft from the harvest site to the back table is where it can be dropped (Fig. 7.6). Everyone on the team must be aware of that potential complication. The options for the dropped graft are to

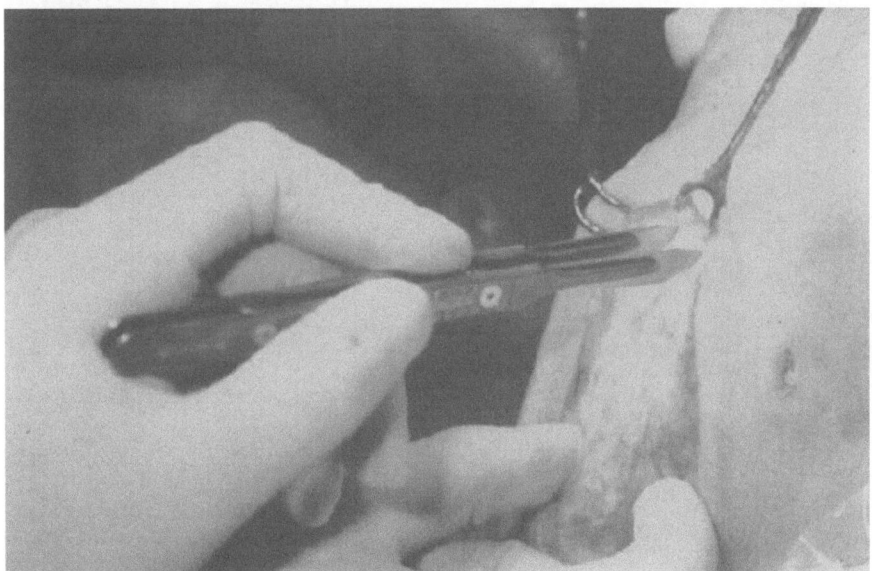

FIGURE 7.4. The harvest of the patellar tendon with a double-bladed knife.

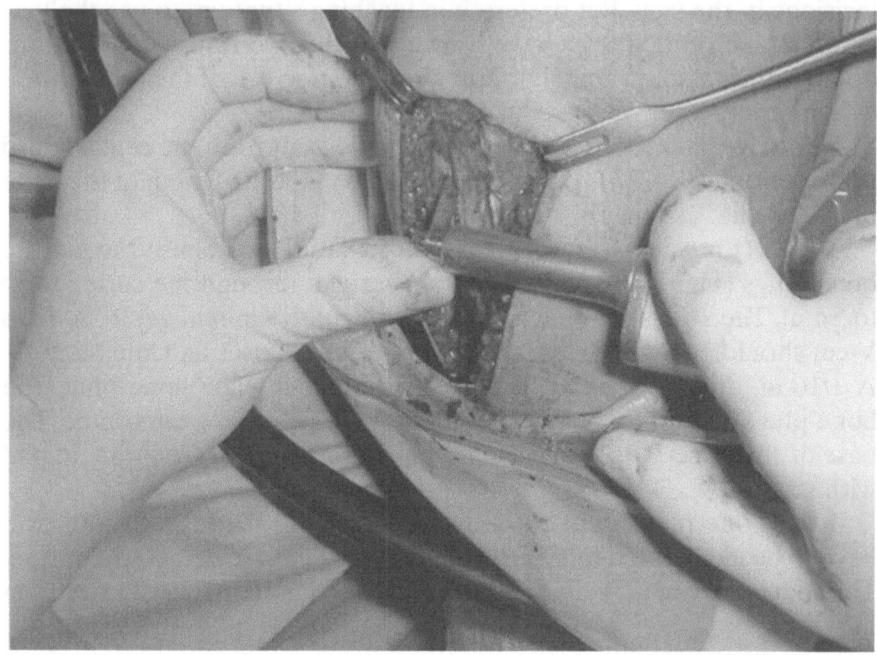

FIGURE 7.5. The patella bone block is cut with the motorized saw.

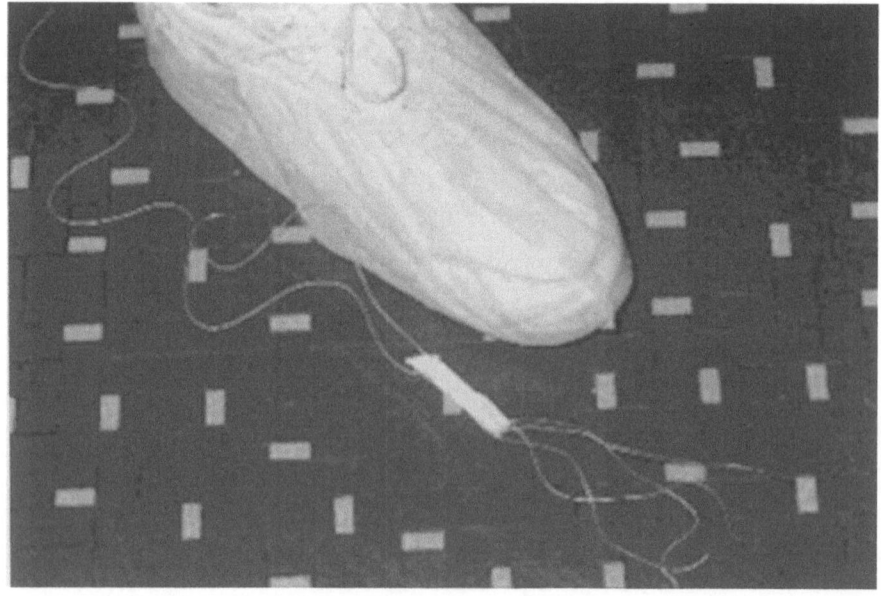

FIGURE 7.6. The dropped graft.

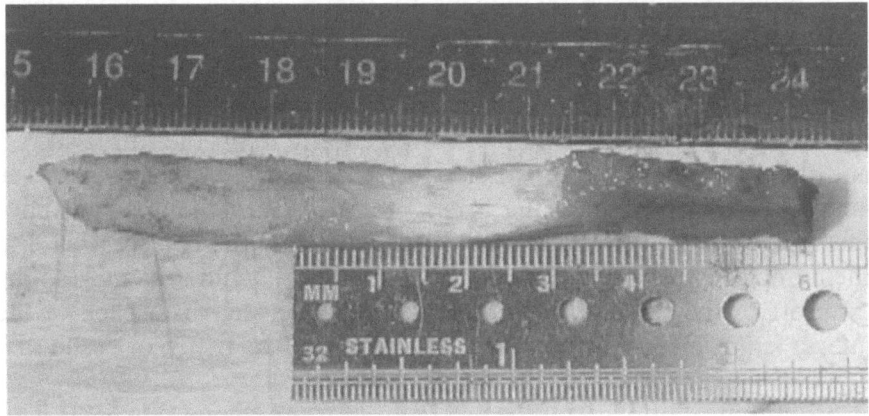

FIGURE 7.7. The patellar tendon graft.

change the graft to semitendinosus, allograft, or synthetic, or to cleanse the graft with chlorhexidine. The cleansing should consist of mechanically irrigating the graft by multiple separate rinsing.

On the back table, the author's group uses a graft preparation table. Measure the total length of the graft (Fig. 7.7). And use a small rongeur or bone cutter to size the bone plugs: the patella plug to 9 mm and the tibia bone plug to 10 mm. The cylindrical sizing tubes from Linvatec should be used to determine the size. The patella end should be made round to pass easily into the femoral tunnel. Leader sutures should be put through the holes in the bone plugs; in the patella use 2 number 0 Vicryl and in the tibia bone plug use 2 number 2 Ti-Cron. The Vicryl sutures (Ethicon, J&J, Boston, MA) are tied together in a knot that rests on the tip of the bone block. This makes it easy to pull into the femoral tunnel. A blue mark with a marking pen is placed at the patella bone tendon junction.

Notchplasty

The lateral wall and roof have to be opened up to accommodate a 10-mm graft. There is still considerable controversy over the notchplasty. Some surgeons do a notchplasty in only 10% of their cases. Others always do one. The author thinks that the answer lies somewhere in between. Each physician should do what must be done to accommodate the graft.

In cases with a very narrow A-frame notch, this will be more extensive (Fig. 6.47). Measure the size of the notch with an instrument, such as a pituitary rongeur that opens to 10 mm. Make the notch large enough to accept this 10-mm instrument. The emphasis should be on the roof and the anterolateral corner. Change the A-shape at the top of the notch to a U-shape. It is important to remove the soft tissue to visualize the back of the notch. I use a large curette to lift the soft tissue off and then a 5.5 mm resector to clean the notch. The critical area to see is the fringe of capsule at the back. The residents ridge does not have this fringe, so the physician should easily identify the correct area. Put the pump pressure at this stage to distend the fat behind the PCL so the drop-off of the femoral condyle can be clearly seen. The back of the lateral femoral condyle has been cleared to see the fringe of tissue that marks the over-the-top position (Fig. 6.50).

A 6-mm oval burr should be used to remove the bone (Fig 6.48). This does not jump around as much as the round burr. Linvatec makes a southpaw for left knees that also eliminates the jumping. The author makes a small divot with the burr at the position that the tunnel should be, that is, 7 mm in from the drop-off, at 11 or 1 o'clock. The major mistake would be not to clear enough soft tissue to expose the posterior aspect of the notch. This can result in drilling the tibial tunnel too anterior. The result is late failure of the graft.

Tibial Tunnel

Figure 6.51 shows the correct external position for the tibial guide. The tip of the Linvatec guide is placed 2-mm medial to the crest of the tibia and 5 cm distal to the joint line. The guide is usually set at 55°. The tip of the guide should be adjacent to the medial collateral ligament. The oblique position will allow the positioning of the femoral guide in an oblique position (Fig. 7.8). The result of this is an oblique graft. This graft position has better long-term stability.

The tip of the guide is in the midline, 7 mm anterior to the PCL (Fig. 6.52). The guide is inserted through the anteromedial portal, by turning it upside down. The knee is flexed to 90°. The surgeon should make sure to aim to bring the long graft passing wire out the anterolateral thigh. The target zone is a 10-cm oval region just above the lateral suprapatellar pouch. Drill a K-wire through the guide into the joint. When the wire hits the guide, loosen it and let the K-wire advance. The guide wire should just touch the leading edge of the PCL (Fig 6.53).

Remove the guide. Ream over the K-wire with a 10 mm drill bit. Clean the interior tunnel site with the 5.5 mm resector. If necessary, chamfer the posterior rim with the chamfering device on the drill. There should be a 3- to 4-mm posterior wall between the tunnel and the PCL

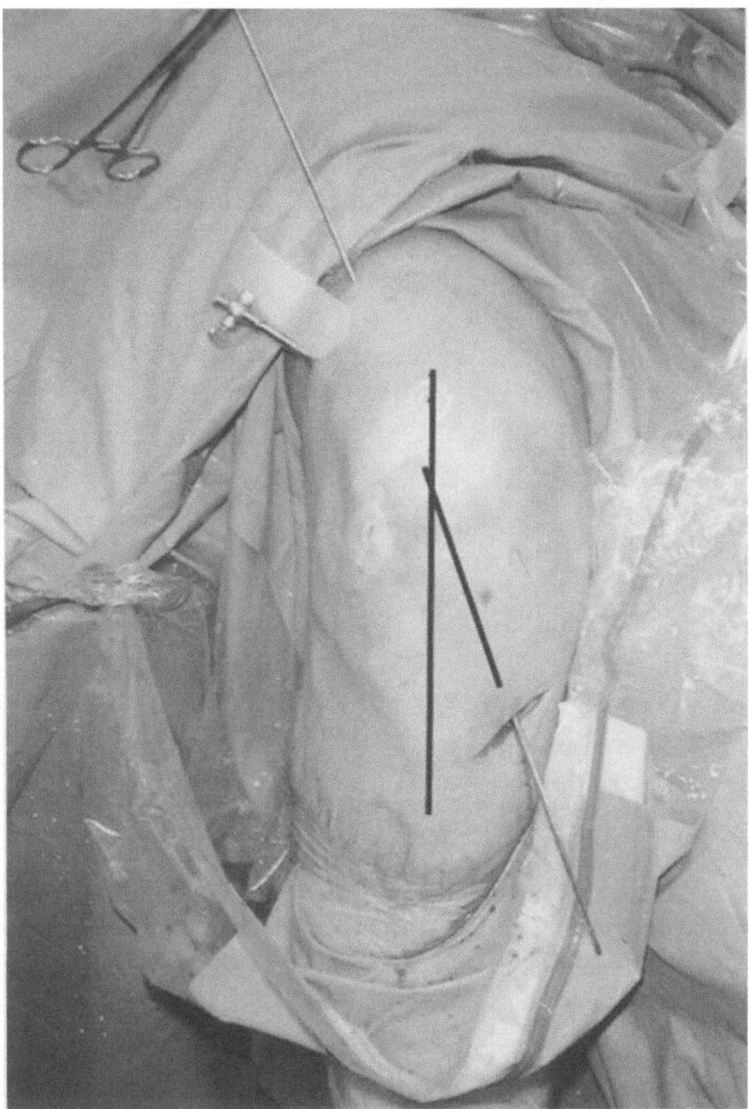

FIGURE 7.8. The oblique position of the tibial tunnel allows the drilling of the femoral tunnel at the 11 or 1 o'clock position.

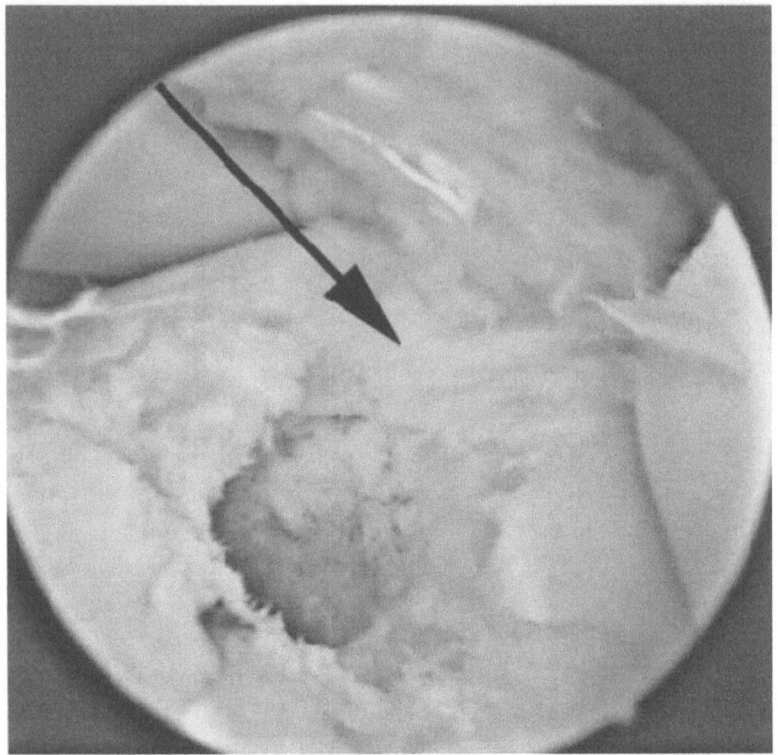

FIGURE 7.9. The position of the tibial tunnel.

(Fig. 7.9). Clean the exterior tunnel site with the 5.5-mm resector. This allows for easy passage of the graft. The video on the CD demonstrates the tunnel procedure.

Femoral Tunnel Patellar Tendon

The Bullseye femoral aiming guide is inserted through the tibial tunnel and hooked over the top of the femur (Fig. 6.54). The femoral tunnel is referenced off the tibial tunnel. The over-the-top Bullseye guide, from the Linvatec GrafFix (Linvatec, Largo, FL) system, is used to position the K-wire for the drill (Fig. 6.55). A K-wire is placed through the guide. The knee should be flexed at 90°. A guide wire should aim for the 11 or 1 o'clock position. This should hit the divot that was marked with the burr earlier. The Bullseye guide is removed and the 10-mm C-reamer is manually advanced to drill the femur (Fig. 6.56). A footprint is drilled deep enough to be sure the posterior cortex is not drilled out. When you have determined that the posterior cortex is intact, advance the bit to a depth of 30 mm (Fig. 6.57). The video on the CD illustrates the procedure. The bit is removed, the K-wire is removed. The knee is flexed to 120°, the notcher inserted into the anteromedial portal, and the supero-lateral aspect of the tunnel is notched (Fig. 6.59). This is the point of insertion of the screw. The notching should only be at the entrance of the tunnel rather than run the whole length. The tunnel is notched to start the BioScrew; avoid breaking the screw in young patients with hard bone.

The eccentric guide is put into the tibial tunnel, through the joint, and again into the tibial tunnel. The two-pin passer is drilled through the eccentric guide (Fig. 7.10). The surgeon should aim for the target zone

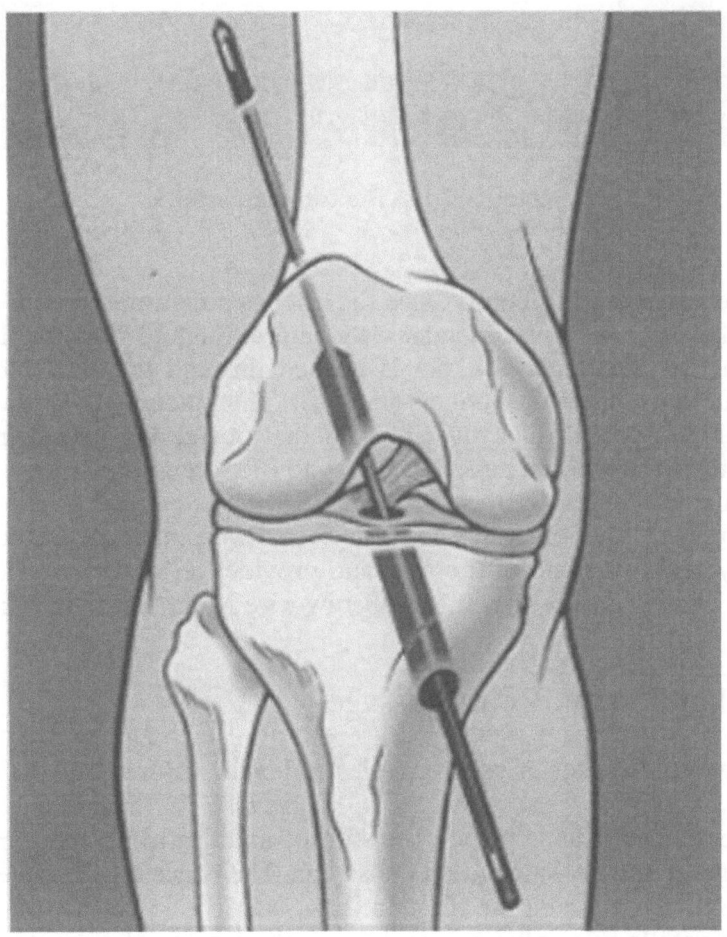

FIGURE 7.10. The two-pin passer.

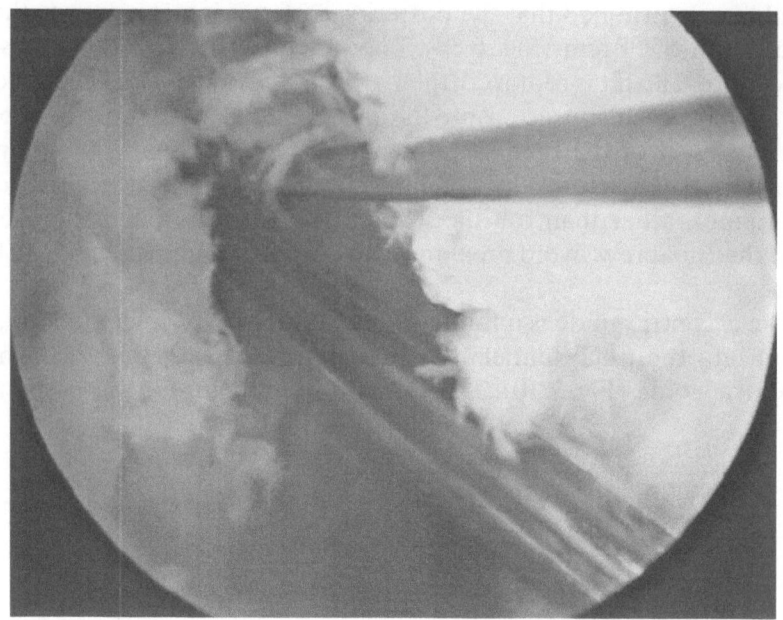

FIGURE 7.11. The two-pin passer.

on the anterolateral femur. Once the pin has penetrated the far cortex, a kocher should be placed against the lateral thigh to stop the pin from skiving up the thigh. The pin is pushed through the skin. Note the oblique position of the tunnels (Fig. 7.8). The guide wire for the screw insertion is put through the anteromedial portal and placed into the channel in the two-pin passer. The second BioScrew guide wire is placed anterior to the graft in the tibia tunnel.

Figure 7.11 demonstrates how the slotted wire pulls the graft up with the eyelet on the end of the wire and provides a slot for the BioScrew guide wire to ensure that the BioScrew wire is parallel to the tunnel.

Patellar Tendon Graft Passage

The two-pin passer is used to pull the leader sutures out the lateral thigh.

The kocher is used to pull the sutures and graft into the joint. The passage should be watched on the screen. The cancellous surface of the graft should be facing the surgeon (Fig. 7.12).

The patella bone plug passes through the intercondylar notch and is pulled into the femoral tunnel. A blue mark is left at the tunnel

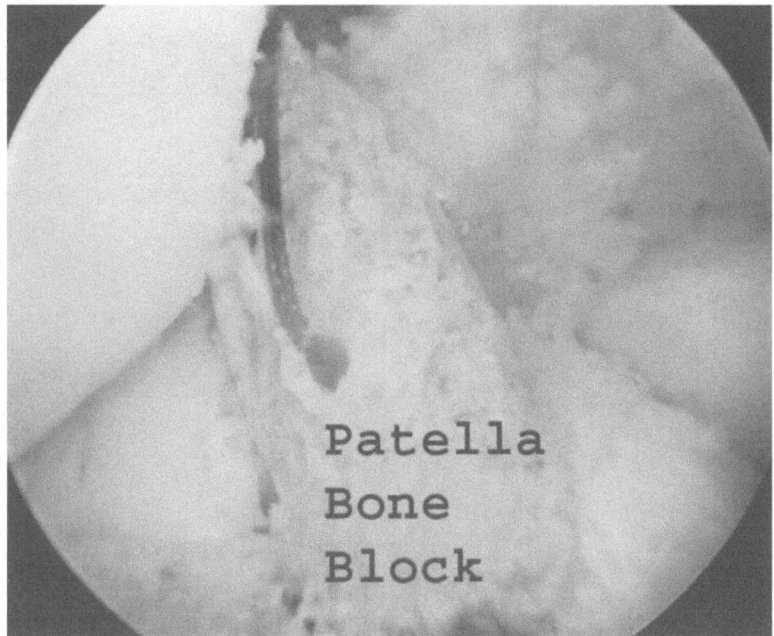

Patella
Bone
Block

FIGURE 7.12. The passage of the patellar tendon graft.

entrance. Tension is maintained on both ends of the leader sutures, and the knee is put through a range of motion to look for adequate clearance in the notch. If there is difficulty in passing the graft, the bone plug may be pulled off. The surgeon will then have to place sutures into the tendon and tie them over a button. The leading edge of the patellar bone plug is tapered like a boat when it is cut. This makes it easier to pass into the femoral tunnel. Remember that the patellar bone plug has also been trimmed to a size of 9 mm, thereby allowing it to pass easily through the 10-mm tunnel.

Graft Fixation

Femoral Fixation

The two-pin passer allows the BioScrew guide wire to be passed directly up the anterior aspect of the femoral tunnel (Fig. 7.13). This avoids kinking of the guide wire when the screw is inserted.

The insertion of the BioScrew should be done with the knee flexed to 120° to avoid injury to the graft and to follow the direction of the

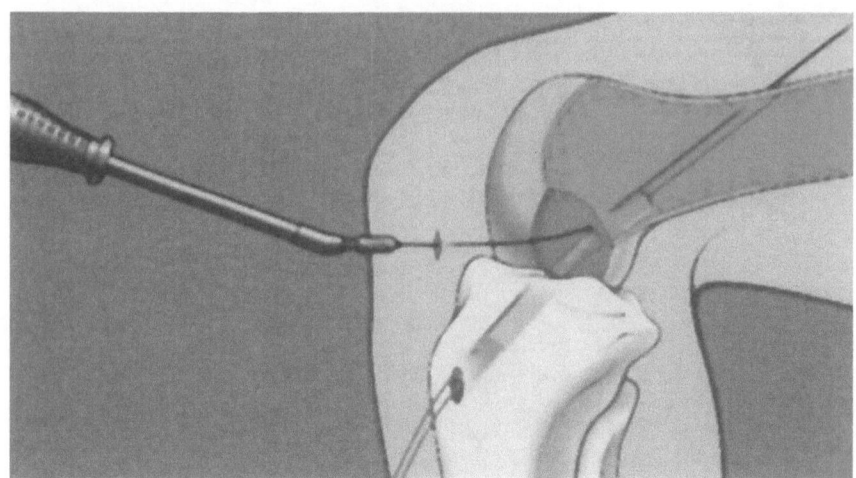

FIGURE 7.13. The two-pin passer.

tunnel (Fig. 6.64). The BioScrew guide wire and the screw should be directed into the notch. Tension is maintained on both sets of leader sutures, and the screw is slowly advanced (Fig. 7.14). Once into the tunnel, the screw will start to squeak, and the surgeon will feel a good purchase in the bone tunnel.

The video on the CD shows how the screw is inserted flush with the tunnel exit and the bone plug. The screw should be against the cancellous side of the bone plug, parallel with the tunnel. This configuration places the tendon in the most posterior aspect of the tunnel. With the BioScrew, the surgeon has one chance to get it right, so do not remove and replace it unless it is necessary to go up a size. The screw should not be forced, as it might break or deform the threads. If it is difficult to start, use the BioScrew tap. The main advantage of the BioScrew is that it will eventually disappear. The author has revised a patellar tendon graft at two years. It was very easy to drill through the remnants of the BioScrew.

Tibial Fixation

The knee is placed at 20° to 30° of flexion, pulling with 12 to 15 lbs on the distal sutures. The smooth K-wire is pushed up the tunnel. Its position is confirmed arthroscopically. An 8 × 25-mm BioScrew is introduced along the K-wire and into the tunnel (Fig. 7.15). Steady tension is maintained on the sutures. Two sutures should be used in the tibial bone plug at slightly different angles. If one suture is cut by the screw insertion,

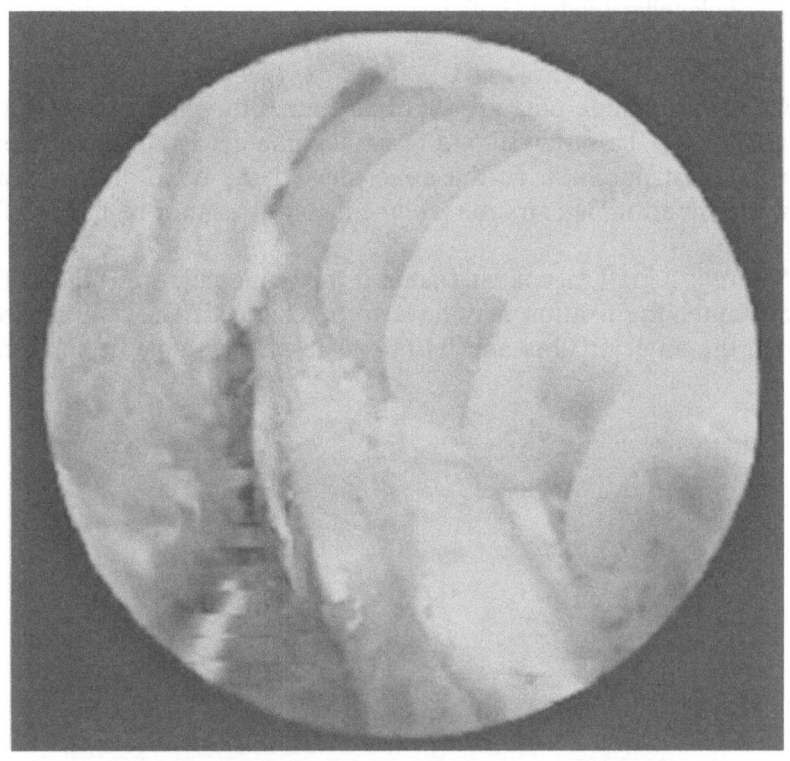

FIGURE 7.14. The insertion of the femoral BioScrew anterior to the graft.

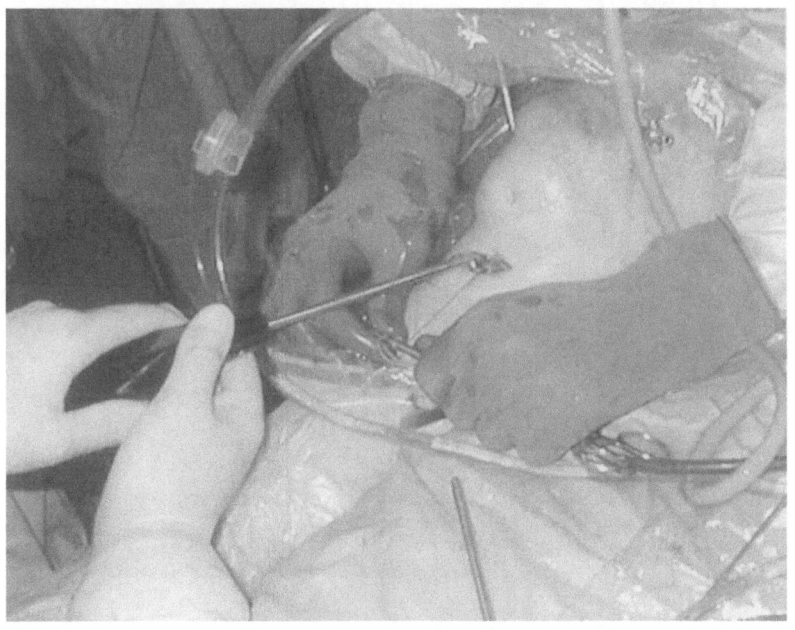

FIGURE 7.15. The insertion of the tibial BioScrew.

the surgeon will always have a backup. Guard against letting the screw push the bone plug up the tibial tunnel by pulling firmly on the distal sutures. The screw should remain at the external tibial cortex to have the best purchase on the bone plug. If the bone plug protrudes from the tibial tunnel, an interference fit screw cannot be used to fix it (Fig. 7.16).

If there is a graft mismatch, that is, if the bone plug protrudes out the tibial tunnel, the fixation may have to be changed. The options are to groove the anterior tibia and fix the graft with a staple or small frag-

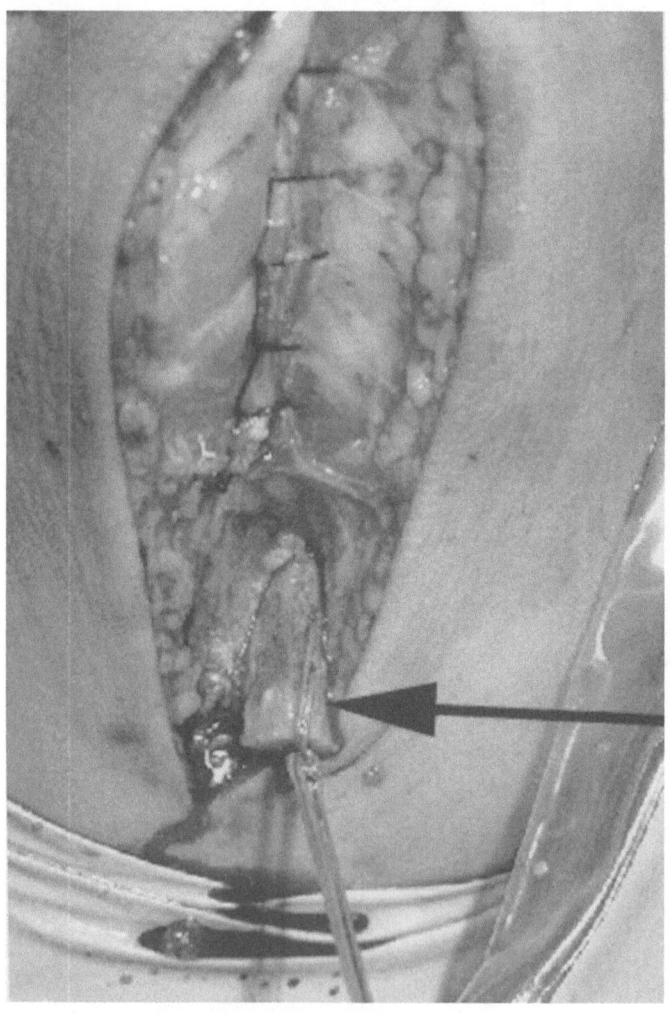

FIGURE 7.16. Graft tunnel mismatch.

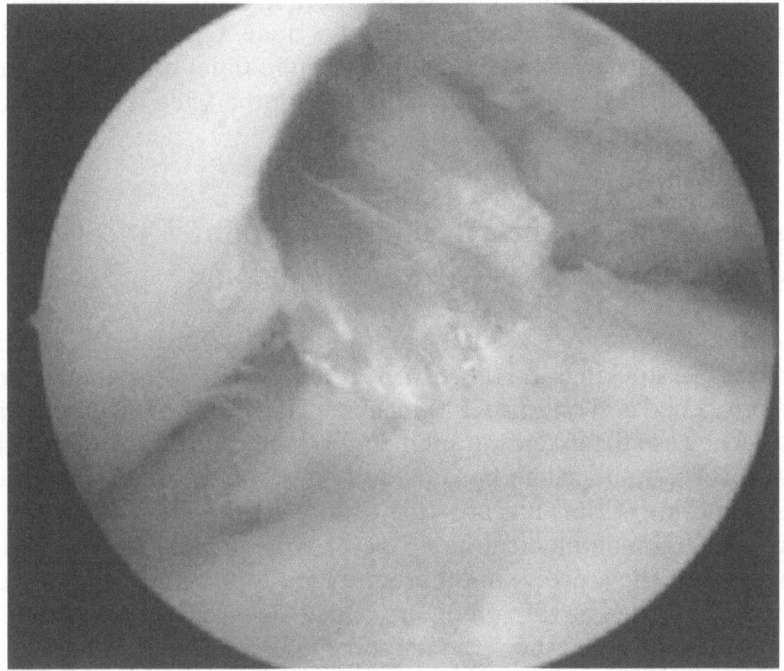

FIGURE 7.17. The completed patellar tendon graft.

ment screw in the groove or to tie the sutures over a screw post placed more distally in the tibia.

Graft Inspection: Look and Hook

Figure 7.17 shows the final inspection of the graft. The graft is inspected as the knee is moved through a range of motion, looking for anterior impingement and lateral wall abrasion. The hook is used to assess tension in the graft. A manual Lachman test is done watching the motion of the tibial spine.

KT-S Measurements

Before the sutures are cut, the KT-S is used to pull a manual maximum a-p translation (Fig. 6.70). This is compared to the normal side. If the other side is not normal, then 5 to 7 mm is taken as normal. Generally the manual maximum will be less than the opposite side. Approximately

10% of the time, the difference is greater than 3 mm, and revision of the tensioning of the graft at the tibial end is done. One common problem is letting the screw push the bone plug up the tibial tunnel. The sutures are cut off when the surgeon is satisfied that the knee is stable and the fixation is secure.

Postoperative Regimen: Extension Splint, Cryo-Cuff, and Continuous Passive Motion Machine

After the wounds are closed, the author applies a Tegaderm dressing, a compressive stocking, and the Cryo-Cuff (Fig. 6.71). The patient is transferred to a bed and on to a CPM machine (Fig. 6.72). When the patients get up, they use the extension splint and crutches (Fig. 6.73). The patient stays several hours in the hospital and goes home with the continuous passive motion (CPM) machine, the Cryo-Cuff, the extension splint, and crutches. Oral pain medication is one or two Tylenol # 3 every 4 hours as necessary. They receive another intravenous dosage of Ancef. Weight bearing is allowed as tolerated. The patient is discharged the same day after several hours in the recovery room.

The patient returns for a checkup in four to five days. The Jones and Tegaderm dressing is removed, and the Cryo-Cuff is applied directly to the skin. The wounds are cleansed for the next few days with 3% hydrogen peroxide. Physiotherapy starts within four to five days. The author has a protocol that can be mailed to remote physiotherapy locations, as well as posted on our Web site, to ensure that the early extension routine is started.

Note that the only difference in the rehabilitation protocol between the semitendinosus and the patellar tendon grafts is that with the semi-t, active knee flexion exercises are avoided for six weeks.

8
Rehabilitation

The patient should have a full understanding of the operative procedure and the postoperative rehabilitation stages. Before the operative procedure, there should be no effusion, a full range of motion, and good quadriceps and hamstring strength.

Postoperative Goals

Physiotherapy should begin the day of surgery if the final result is to be full range of motion, no effusion, and strength equal to the opposite side. Individuals will vary in their progress on this program. The surgeon or physiotherapist should make any necessary alterations in this program.

It is important that there be only closed-kinetic chain-type exercises. That means the quadriceps should be actively exercised when the joint is weight bearing. Avoid active leg extensions in the last 30° when sitting. For the hamstring graft, there should be no active resisted knee flexion exercises for six weeks. This allows the muscle harvest site to heal.

This protocol may need to be modified according the type of fixation used and if additional surgery is performed to the MCL, LCL, or because of meniscal repair. The exercise program may be reviewed on the video on the CD.

Day 1

Goal

- Decrease pain and swelling.

Ambulation

- The patient may be able to tolerate partial weight bearing with a Zimmer splint (Fig. 6.73).

- The extension splint must be worn while sleeping (if patient is using CPM, the splint is removed) (Fig. 6.72).

Exercises and Activities

- For the first few days the patient should rest, with the knee elevated on the CPM machine and Cryo-Cuff or ice pack used continuously.
- Isometric quadriceps exercises may be done (Fig. 6.71).

Days 2 to 14

Goals

- To obtain full extension or hyperextension.
- To minimize swelling.
- To allow wound healing.
- To maintain active quads control.
- To achieve 90° of flexion.

Ambulation

- The patient may tolerate weight bearing with a Zimmer splint.
- By day 7, the patient should be full weight bearing using only the splint.
- The extension splint must be worn at night until full extension is obtained.
- Walking should be minimized to decrease swelling of the leg.
- The extension splint may be removed for exercise on the CPM and for bathing, sitting, and resting.
- When the wounds have healed, the functional knee brace may be used rather than the extension splint.

Exercises and Activities

- Passive knee extensions are performed with ice, and the heel on a block (Fig. 8.1).
- Passive knee flexion is performed by doing wall slides (Fig. 8.2).
- Quadriceps static sets are done with the patient in the sitting position and with a towel under the heel. Electrical muscle stimulation can be performed at the same time (Fig. 8.3).
- Gastrocnemius stretches are done with a towel around the foot. This also encourages knee extension (Fig 8.4).

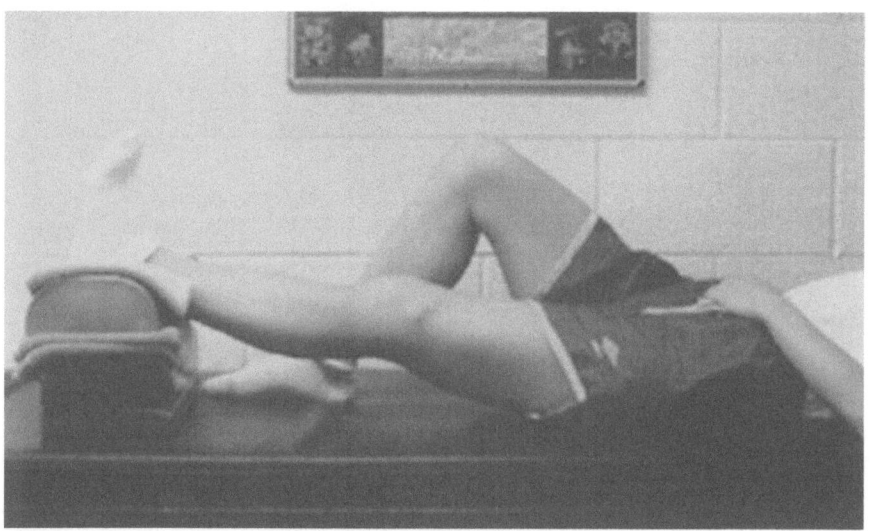

FIGURE 8.1. Passive knee extension.

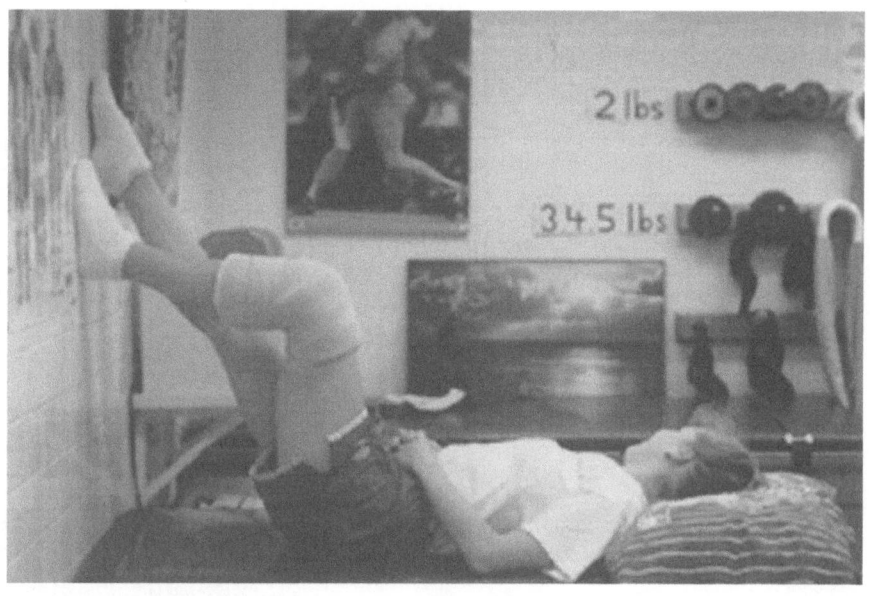

FIGURE 8.2. Wall slides for passive knee flexion.

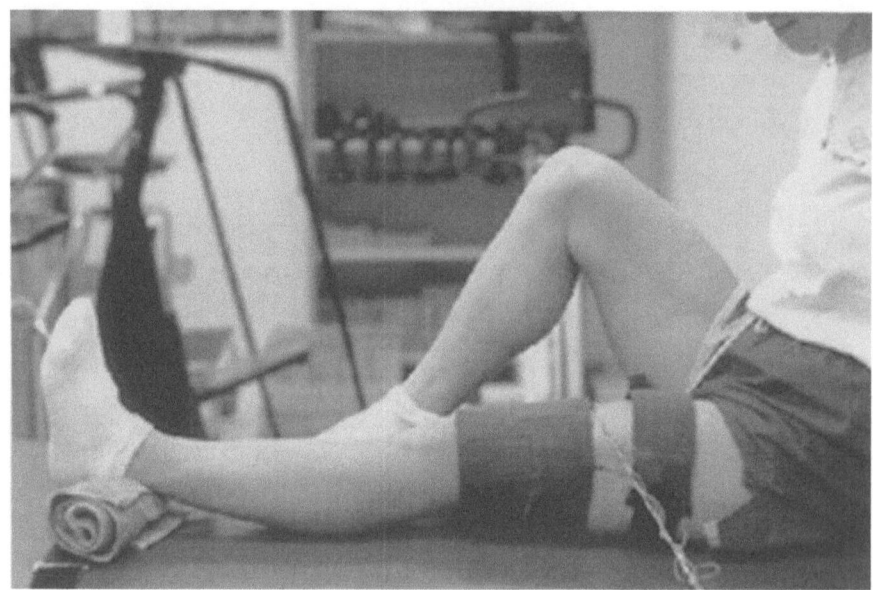

FIGURE 8.3. Electrical muscle stimulation.

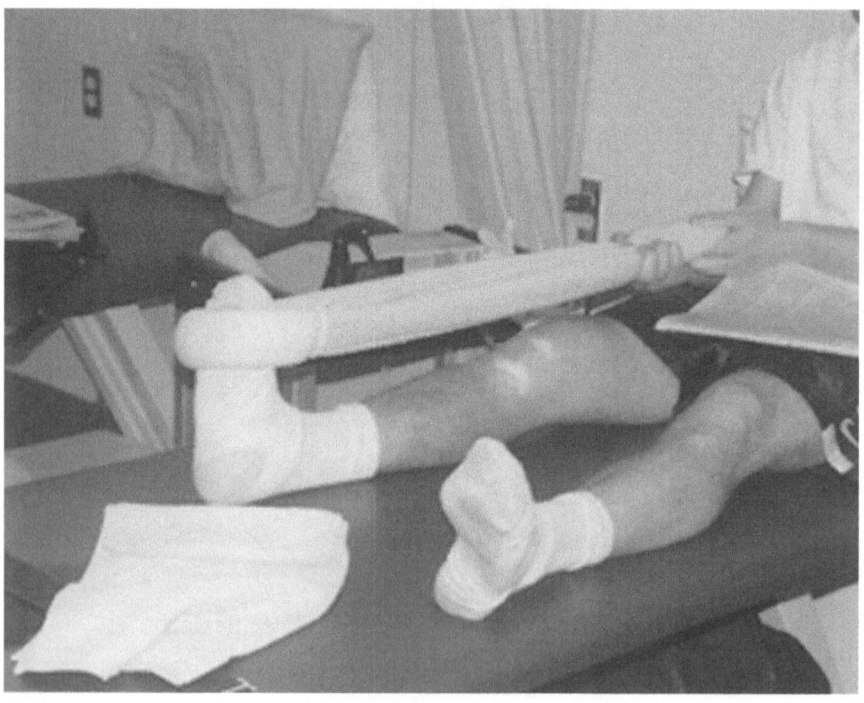

FIGURE 8.4. Gastrocnemius stretch with towel.

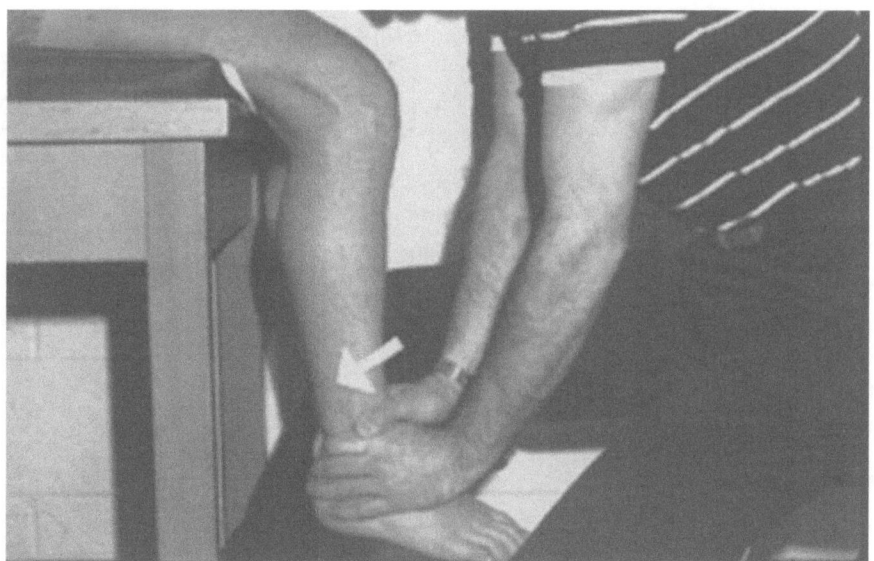

FIGURE 8.5. Passive flexion.

- Isometrics: Multirange of 90° to 60° (not beyond 60°), using Thera-Band or opposite leg.
- Quad set: Standing against wall, pushing back extending knee into rolled towel, progressing to straight leg raising to 30° in standing position.
- Passive flexion over the edge of the bed may be augmented by traction by the therapist (Fig. 8.5).
- Patellar mobilizations are performed by the therapist if the patellar mobility is becoming limited. (Fig. 8.6).
- Hip adductors/abductors strengthening as tolerated.
- Hamstrings: Active progress to resisted. (Do not do if hamstring reconstruction has been performed.)
- Heel raises.
- Proprioceptive exercises can be done by standing on the surgical leg, progressing to stork lifting free leg in front and behind or by using a rocker board (Fig. 8.7).

Weeks 2 to 6

Goals

- To increase flexion to 135°.
- To decrease swelling.
- To increase muscle tone.

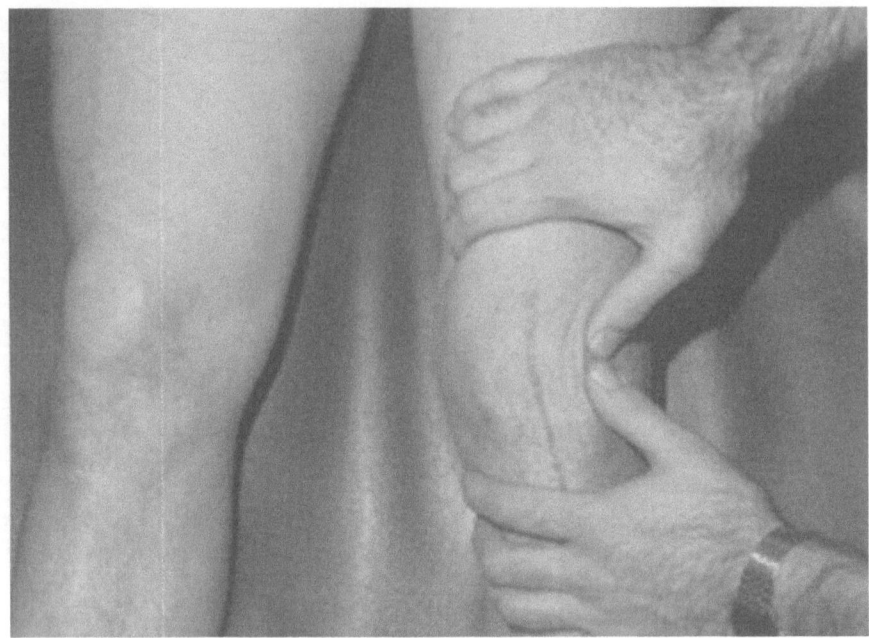

FIGURE 8.6. Patellar mobilizations.

Ambulation

- The patient should tolerate full weight bearing with the extension splint or the functional DonJoy Brace. The splint may be discontinued at home.

Exercises and Activities

- Quadriceps exercises: Straight leg raising in supine (only if no quads lag).
- Double leg: Progress to single leg squat (to 45° flexion).
- Hamstrings: If lack of full extension, start prone hangs with weight.
- The step up and step down exercise is performed initially with 4-in. blocks and progresses to a 6-in. block (Fig. 8.8).
- Stair climber: Progress slowly (Fig. 8.9).
- The stationary bike is used to increase range of motion and muscle strength (Fig. 8.10).
- Swimming: If incisions are healed, begin with forward and backward walking in water. Use buoy between the knees to swim or use the dolphin kick.
- Progress proprioception from bilateral to single leg wobble board, no rotation.

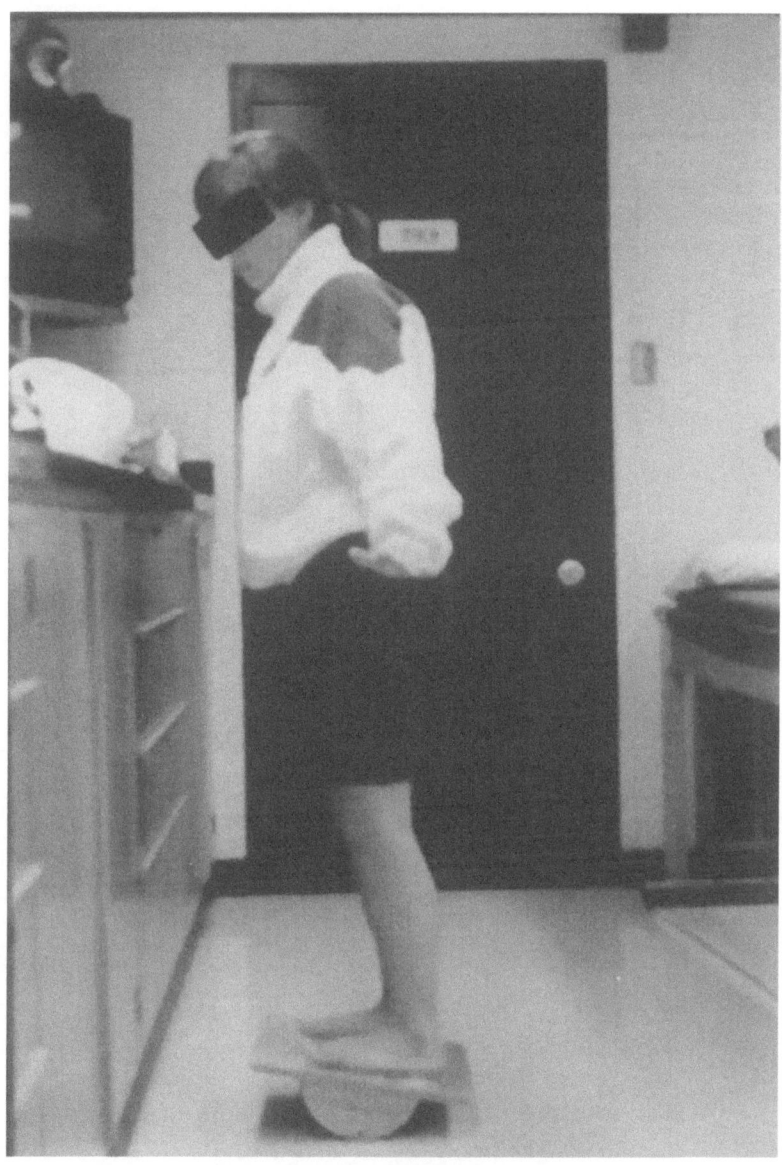

FIGURE 8.7. Proprioceptive exercises.

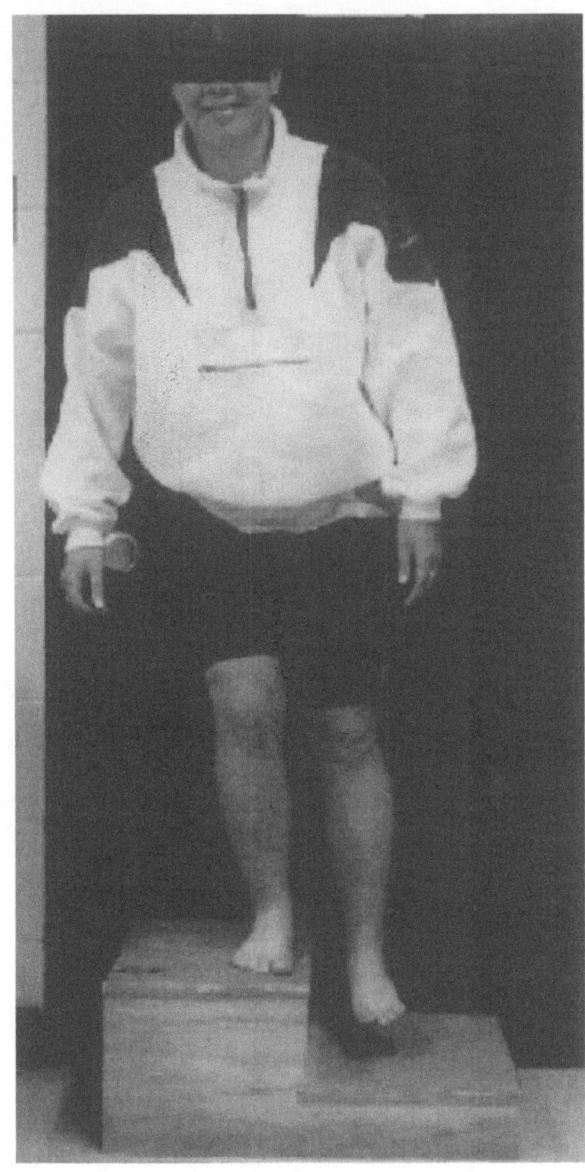

FIGURE 8.8. Block steps.

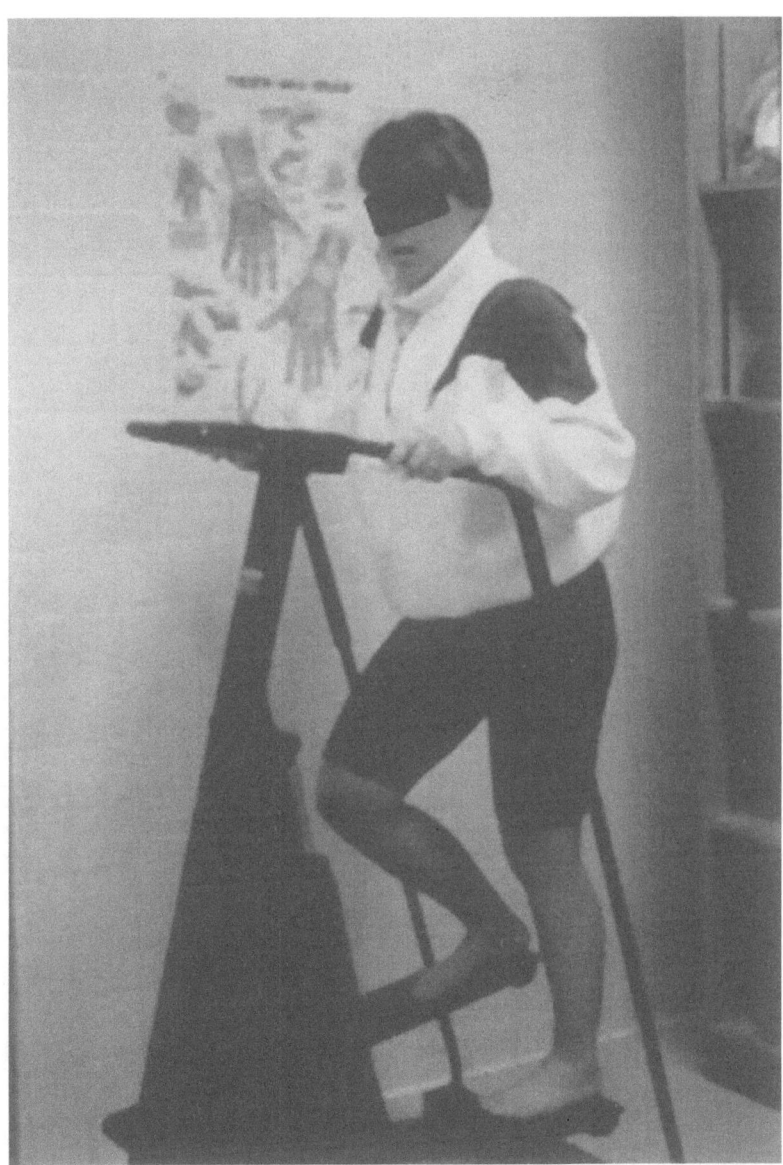

FIGURE 8.9. Stair climber: progress slowly.

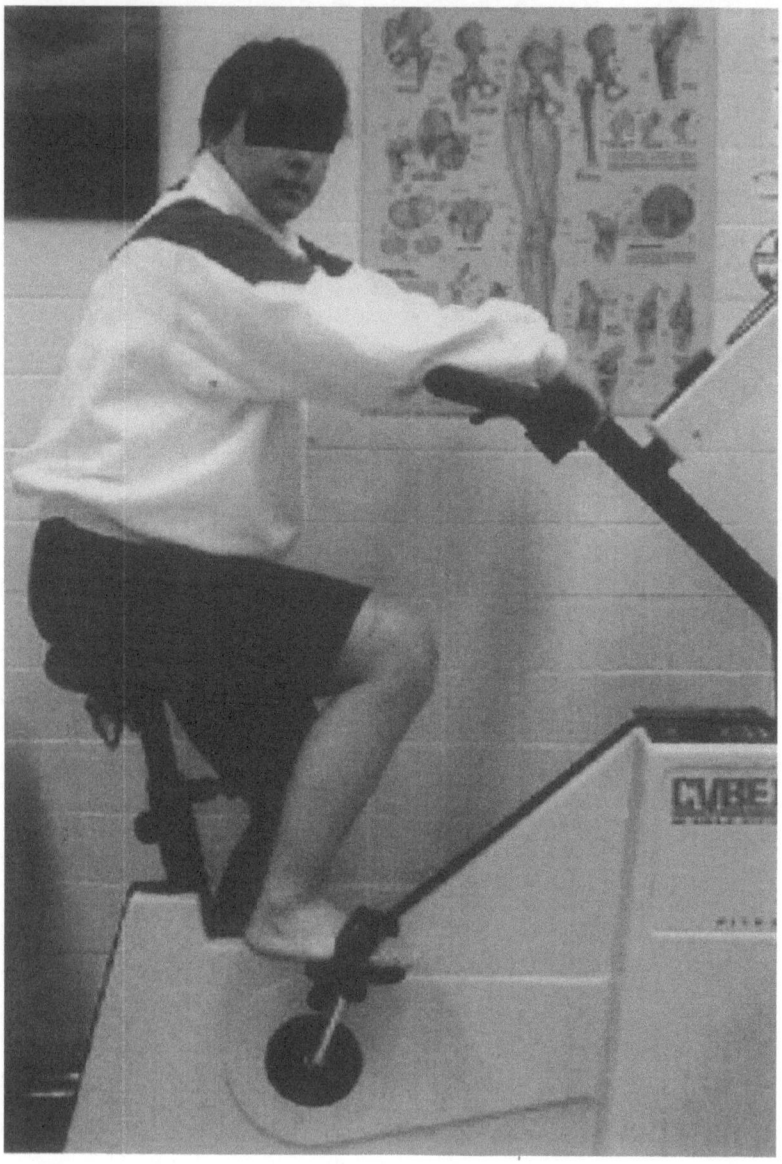

FIGURE 8.10. Stationary bike.

- Hip rotators with Thera-Band. (Do not use if collateral ligament repair.)

Weeks 6 to 9

Goals

- To progress to full range of motion
- To increase strength
- To increase functional activities.

Ambulation

- The patient should be full weight bearing without the splint, but should continue the functional brace when active.

Exercises and Activities

- Swimming: Add flutter kick at poolside or flutter board. Progress to front crawl/back crawl if comfort permits.
- Easy jogging in waist-deep water.
- Cycle outdoors on level terrain, with no toe clips or standing.
- Power walking.
- Hamstring reconstruction patients may start hamstring-resisted exercises.

Weeks 9 to 12

Goals

- To increase functional activities
- To improve muscle strength and endurance.

Ambulation

- Full weight bearing.

Exercises and Activities

- Progress power walking to walk/jog on level surface.
- Lunges.
- Cycling on all types of terrain.
- Phantom chair: Begin at 45° and progress to 90°.

- Cybex isokinetic exercises may be started with antishear device.
- Skipping: Both legs.

Weeks 12+

Goals

- To maintain the full range of motion.
- To increase function, strength, and endurance.

Ambulation

- Full weight bearing.

Exercises and Activities

- Muscle strengthening exercises for both the quads and hamstrings can be done in the gym (Fig. 8.11).
- Leg press and bench squats can also be done.
- Straight ahead running at half speed on level terrain.
- Running up stairs/walking down stairs.
- Introduce interval training on bike.
- Proprioception on balance board and strength program in gym.
- Hopping drills: Progress from two legs to one leg. Work in all directions. Gradually increasing height and/or distance of hops. Then add plyometrics (i.e., hopping down from stairs/boxes).

Week 14+

Exercises and Activities

- Light sport activities (cross-county skiing, curling, golf, ice skating) may be started only if there is no effusion and there is a full range of motion and 75% quad/ham strength ratio (85% for roller blading), a negative Lachman test, and physician approval (Fig 8.12).

Months 6+

Exercises and Activities

- Vigorous pivoting activities may be resumed if the reconstructed knee is 90% of the strength of the opposite knee.

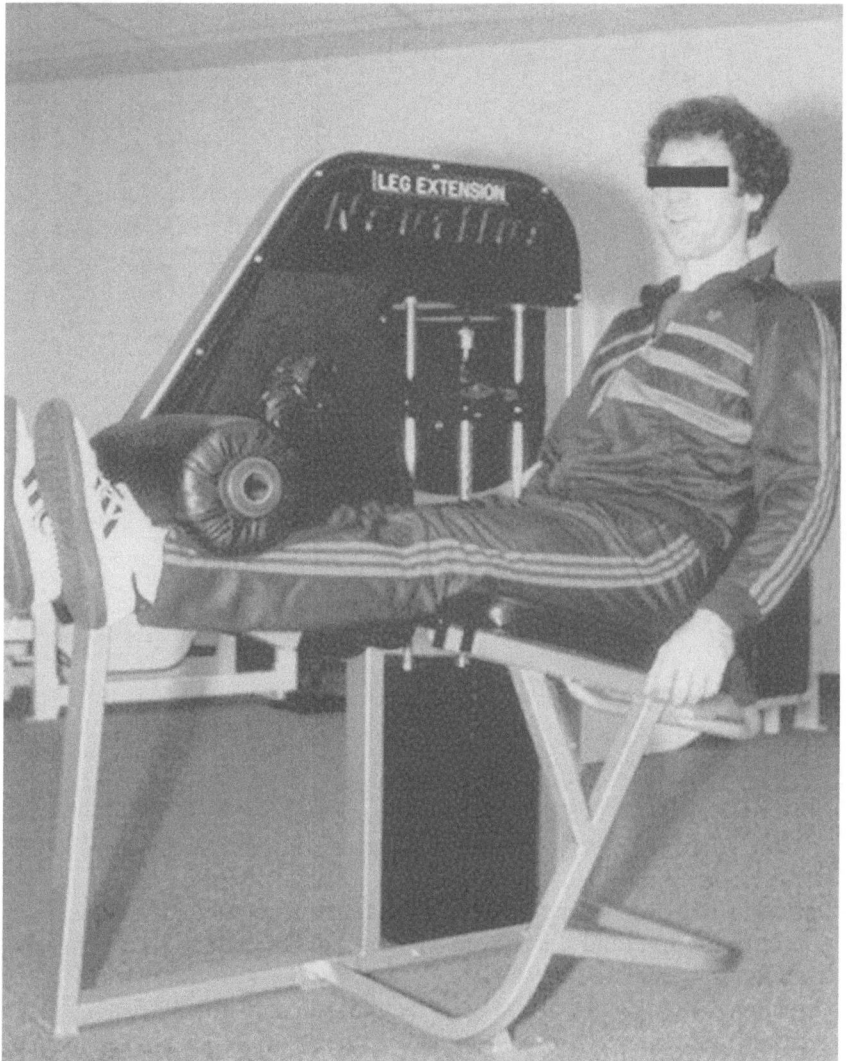

FIGURE 8.11. Progressive resisted exercises in the gym.

- It is advisable to wear the functional knee brace for first year post-operatively. The use of the brace may be discontinued when the patient has confidence in the knee. This may take as long as 18 months.
- Lateral and pivotal exercises may be started. Start figure-eight exercises with large, lazy eights and then decrease the eight in size and

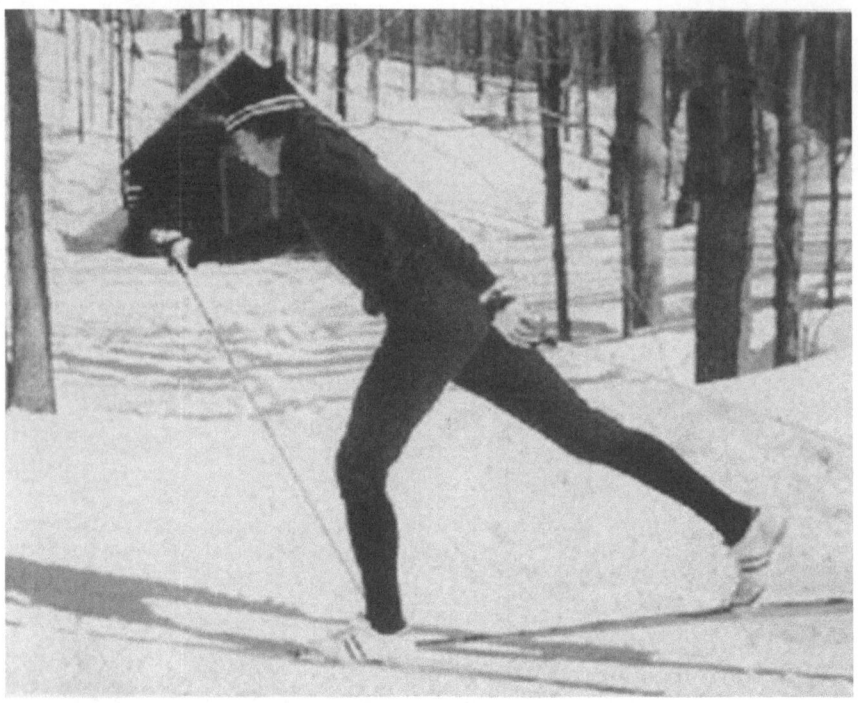

FIGURE 8.12. Outdoor sports such as cross-country skiing.

increase speed (start with 50 m, then progress 30 m, and finally 10 m) (repeat each 10 times).

- Carioca: Running sideways. Cross the left foot in front of and behind right foot for 10 m and then reverse pattern and direction (repeat 5 to 10 times in each direction).
- Directional run: Facing the same direction, run forward, sideways, backward, and sideways, 10 m in a square (repeat 5 to 10 times in each direction).
- Run: Cut 90° running half speed, go 20 m and make a 90° cut to the right, and then repeat to the left (repeat 10 to 20 times in each direction).

Modifications to Protocol

- ACL and LCL repairs: Avoid varus stress by wearing the protective functional brace for six months.

- ACL and MCL repairs: Avoid valgus stress wearing the protective functional brace for six months.
- ACL and PCL: Modify the protocol and brace in extension for six weeks.
- ACL and meniscal repairs: Follow the ACL protocol. The only restriction is no full weight-bearing squats for six weeks.

9
Complications

Everyone is eventually going to have a complication with ACL reconstruction; it is just a matter of how serious the problem will be. It is
important to realize the potential problems: How to deal with them and
how to avoid them. No one likes complications, but the surgeon who is
prepared to deal with them will rise above the others. Remember, it is
not if, but when, and how bad the complications will be. The format of
the discussion will be to present the problem, give a solution to the
problem, and finally offer a prevention for the problem.

Preoperative Considerations

Patient Selection

The noncompliant patient who returns to sport too quickly may be at
risk to rupture the weak graft. The opposite type of patient, that is, the
nervous, anxious, or extremely apprehensive patient, is at risk to develop
stiffness. If these patient profiles are recognized, appropriate preventive
measures can be taken.

Anterior Knee Pain

Problem

Preoperative anterior knee pain may indicate use of the hamstring graft.
Avoiding any trauma to the patellofemoral joint is advisable in patients
with patellofemoral syndrome.

Solution

Avoid the patellar tendon graft. Modify the rehabilitation program to
avoid any concentric-resisted quadriceps exercises. The weight program
may have to be eliminated entirely, and the exercise bike, with toe
straps, may be the only form of activity tolerated.

Prevention

Daniel stated that the principal cause of anterior knee pain is the lack of extension. He felt that the flexion contracture led to increased patellofemoral contact force and to the development of chondromalacia patella. The aggressive rehabilitation program that emphasizes early knee extension may prevent the development of the flexion contracture.

Timing of Operation

The acute knee, with a marked limited range of motion, and induration, should be treated conservatively, until the knee becomes less inflamed. Operation in this acute situation often results in postoperative stiffness and difficulty in obtaining range of motion.

Immature Athlete

The preteenage athlete with an ACL tear is a rare clinical situation, and is difficult to manage. The natural history of the immature athlete with an ACL tear is pessimistic. If the youngster cannot, or will not, give up sports, then an ACL reconstruction should be carried out. The objective is to stabilize the knee and prevent recurrent giving way episodes that cause further damage to the meniscus and the articular surface. The operation should avoid injury to the epiphysis. The tibial tunnel should be drilled in the center of the epiphysis, avoiding the tibial tubercle. The semitendinosus graft should be taken over the top or through a femoral tunnel and fixed with an Endo-button. With these precautions, injury to the growth plate is rare. In the preoperative assessment of the teenager, it is important to X-ray the patient to assess the growth plates around the knee.

Medial Compartment Osteoarthritis and the ACL-Deficient Knee

The association of medial compartment osteoarthritis and the ACL-deficient knee is a common clinical situation. In the early phase, the ACL reconstruction should be the principal procedure, with an arthroscopic debridement of the medial compartment.

When the medial compartment wear is more severe, and the patient is still complaining of giving way, still has a positive pivot-shift test, and has a moderate degree of clinical varus in the standing position, then the ligament reconstruction should be combined with a high tibial osteotomy.

When the medial compartment wear is marked, the varus is moderately severe, the patient lacks full knee extension, and has a negative pivot-shift test, then the high tibial osteotomy should be the only procedure carried out.

Intraoperative Complications

Patellar Tendon Harvest

Problem

The patellar tendon harvest results in a small, thin, or fractured bone plug.

Solution

The first solution is to use a coring reamer in the tibia, and bone graft the plug in a piggyback fashion (Fig. 9.1).

The second solution is to reverse the graft. Use Krackow sutures on the tendon end and tie these over a button (Fig. 9.2). A supplemental, large BioScrew may be used to secure the tendon in the tibial tunnel.

Prevention

The prevention of this complication is to use a saw, such as a cast saw, to initially cut the cortex at 90°, and then cut at a 60° angle to a depth of 8mm (Fig. 9.3). Avoid a deep V-cut to prevent a longitudinal patella fracture. Gently lift out the bone plug with an osteotome. The base should be flat and the top end should be bullet shaped.

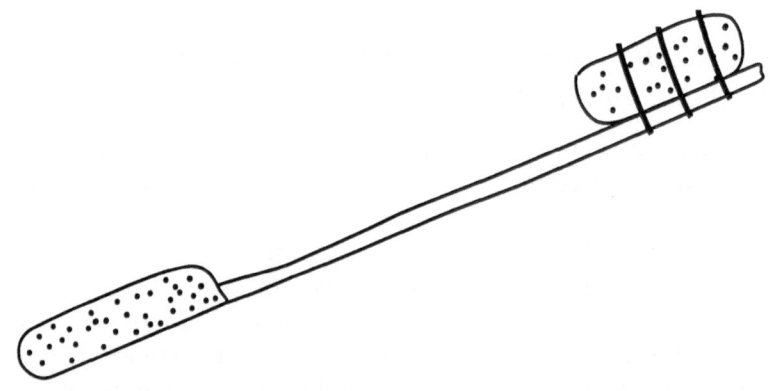

FIGURE 9.1. The bony augmentation of the graft.

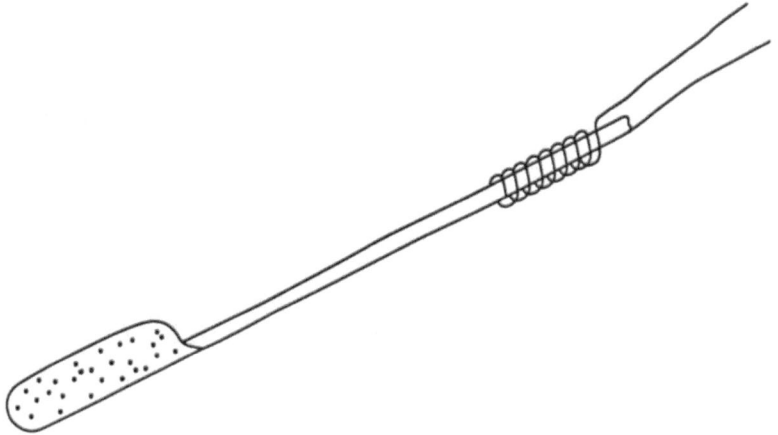

FIGURE 9.2. Suturing of the tendon end of the graft.

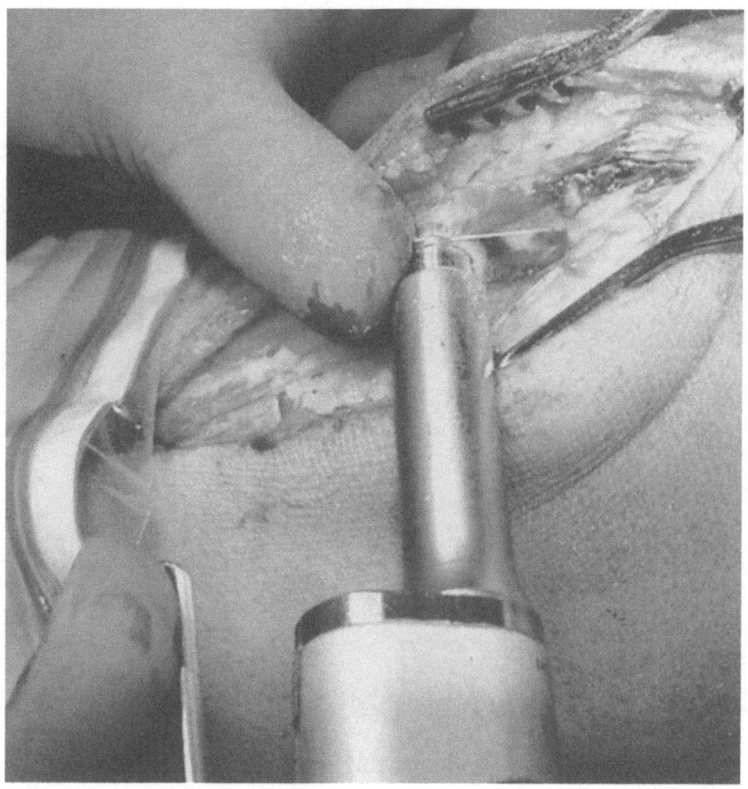

FIGURE 9.3. Cutting the patellar bone plug.

Semi-t Graft Harvest

Problem

The tendon is cut off short. Figure 9.4 shows the amputated tendon that was caused by not cutting the bands to the gastrocnemius before attempting to strip the tendon.

Solution

The graft source may be changed to either a patellar tendon or an allograft. The small piece of graft may be augmented with the gracilis.

Prevention

The short graft may be prevented with a careful harvest technique that emphasizes the cutting of the bands to the gastrocnemius. Figure 9.5 shows the bands to the gastrocnemius that must be cut to advance the stripper up the tendon. When pulling on the tendon, look at the skin over the gastrocnemius for dimpling. If the skin dimples, then the bands have not all been cut. Do not try to advance the stripper in this situa-

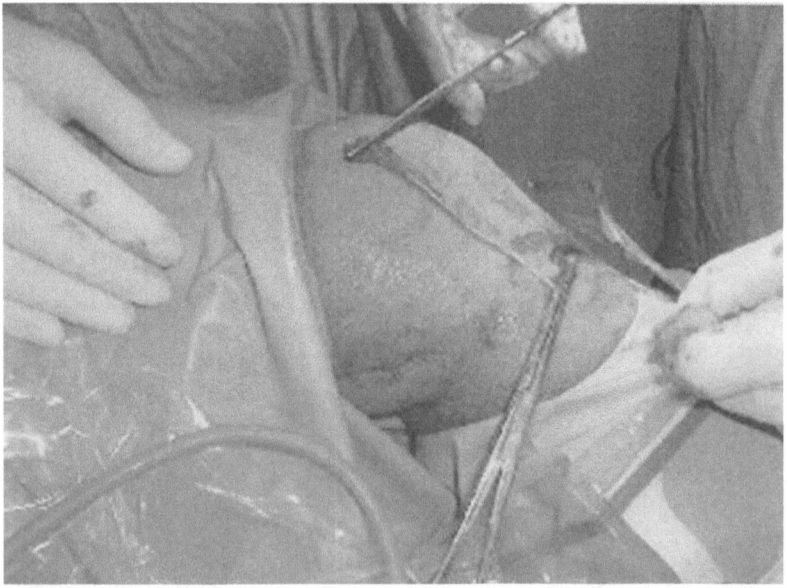

FIGURE 9.4. The hamstring graft is cut off short.

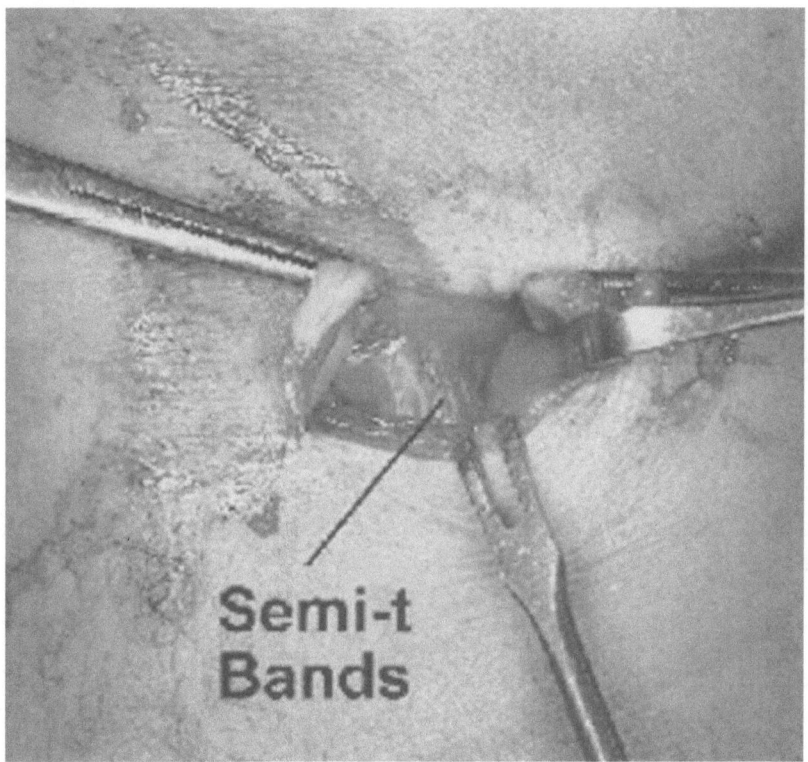

FIGURE 9.5. The bands to the gastrocnemius.

tion. Figure 9.6 demonstrates what happens when the band is not cut, and the stripper is advanced against the band. The tendon becomes kinked and may be cut off short.

Dropped Graft

Problem

The dropped graft is illustrated in Figure 9.7.

Solution

The first option is to change the dropped graft to another graft source, such as the semitendinosus or patellar tendon from the same side. The second option is to cleanse the graft with Hibiclens (chlorhex-

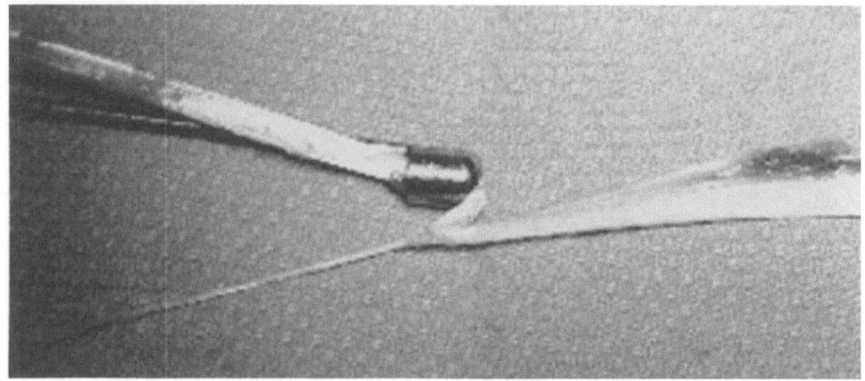

FIGURE 9.6. The band kinks the tendon.

idine). The cleansing should consist of multiple washing and irrigations of the graft.

Prevention

The graft should only be passed with towel clip in a basin (Fig. 9.8). Do not touch the graft. Watch out for the tendon sticking to a glove

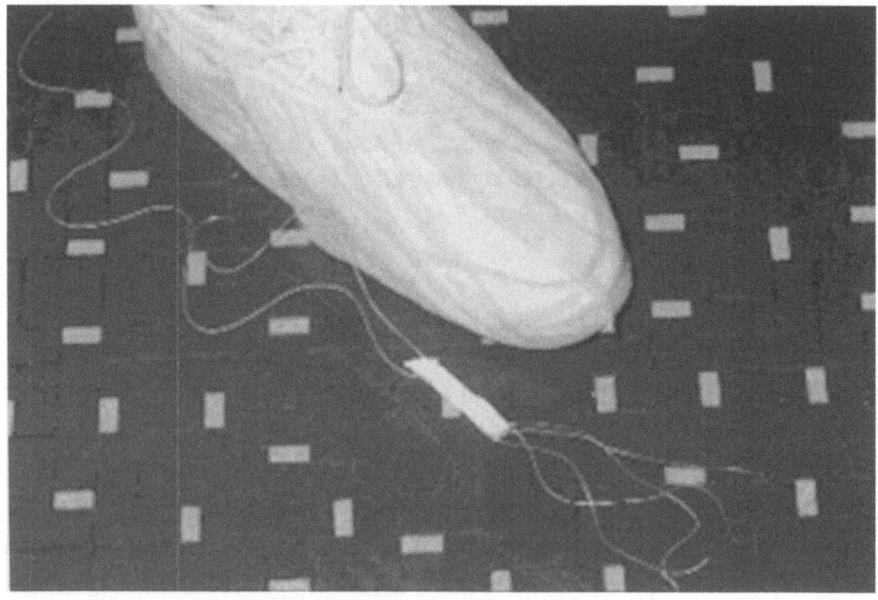

FIGURE 9.7. The dropped graft.

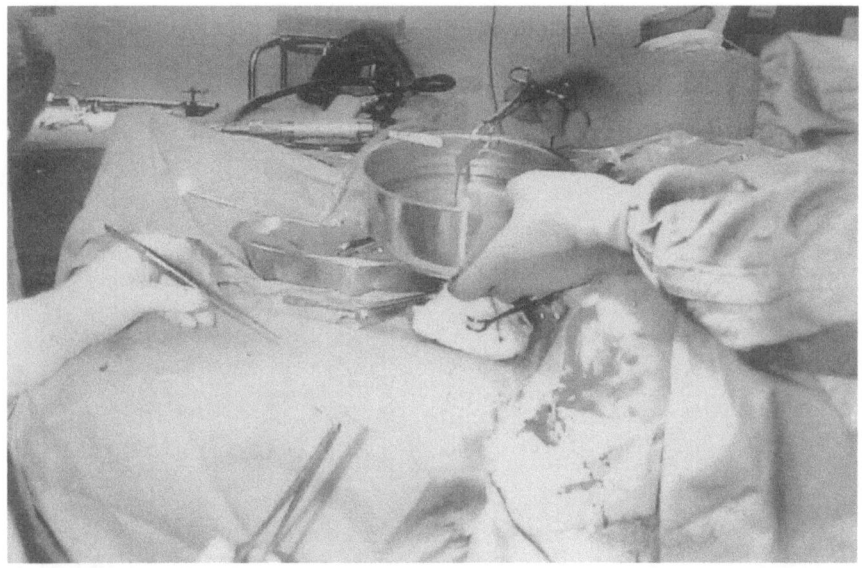

FIGURE 9.8. The tendon is passed in a bowl.

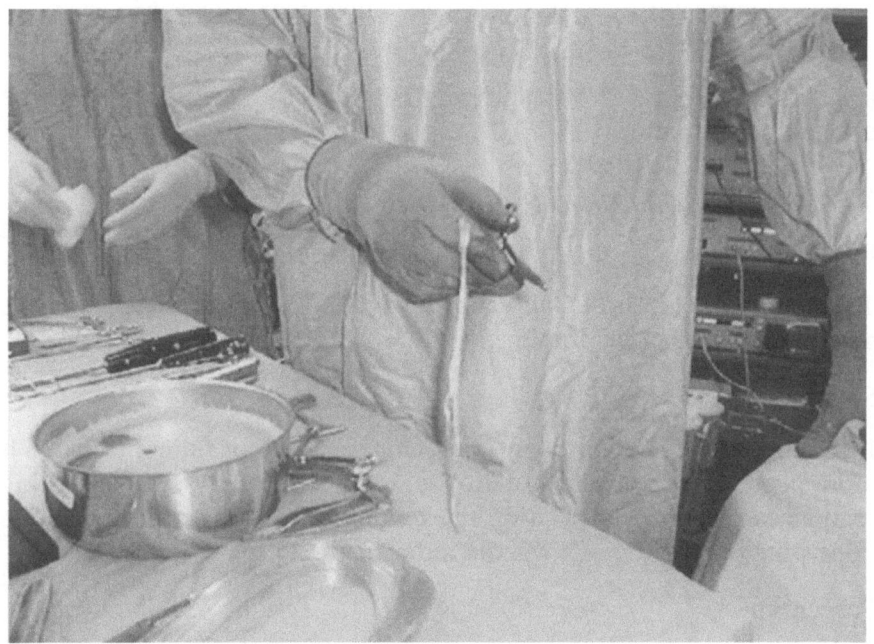

FIGURE 9.9. The tendon can stick to the glove.

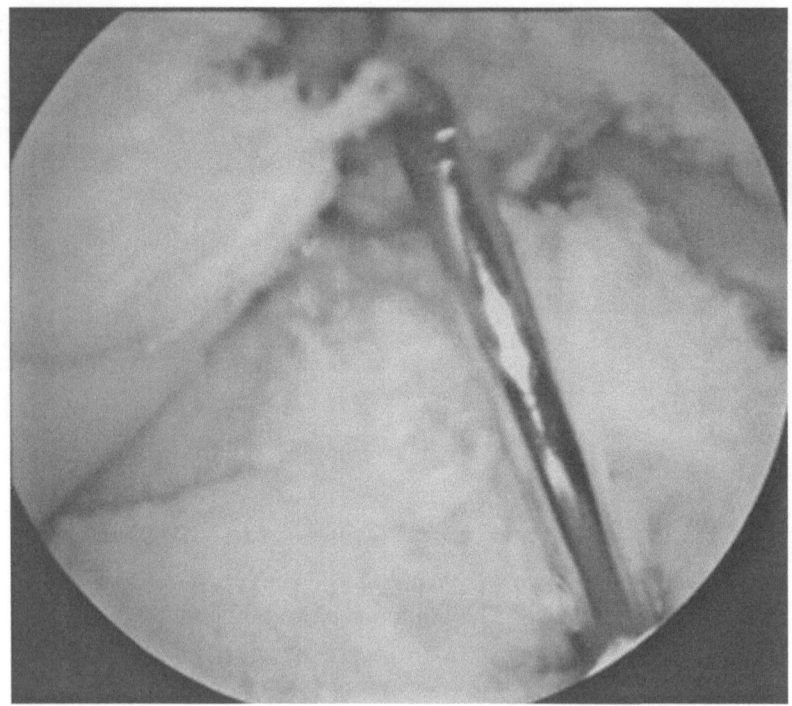

FIGURE 9.10. The anteriorly placed tibial tunnel guide wire.

(Fig. 9.9). It always drops half way between the back table and the operating room table.

Tunnel Malposition: Tibial Tunnel Anterior

Problem

The tibial tunnel is drilled anterior (Fig 9.10). The result is failure of the graft by anterior notch impingement.

Solution

If the tunnel is just slightly anterior, chamfer back of tunnel to move it more posterior. The usual situation is similar to Figure 9.10. The coring reamer can be used to position the tunnel in the correct position. The bone plug is used to graft the old anterior tunnel.

Prevention

Before drilling the tunnel, use a K-wire and if necessary reposition the wire to the correct position before drilling the tunnel. Always check the

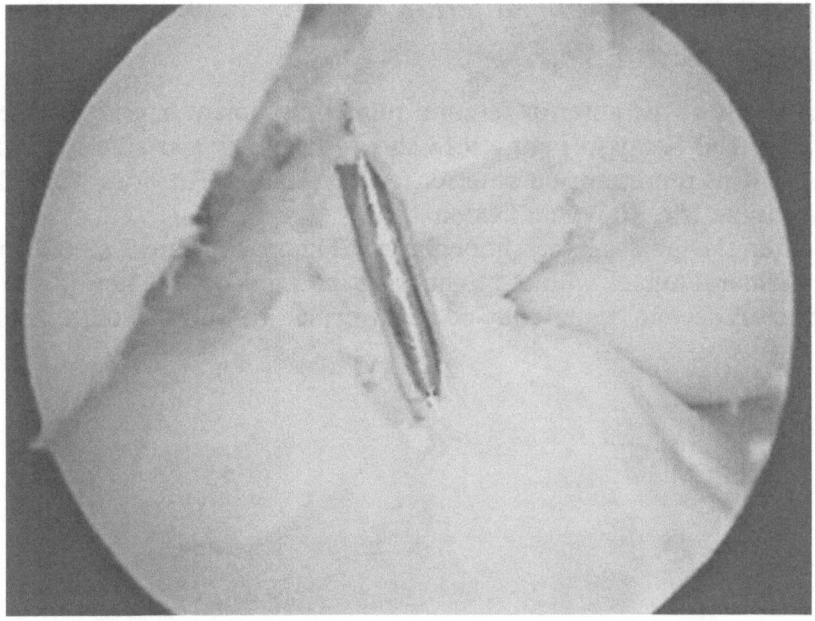

FIGURE 9.11. The correct position for the tibial guide wire.

wire position by extending the knee with the K-wire in the notch to see if there is enough clearance for the graft in the notch. Use the landmarks to position the wire, 7 mm anterior to the PCL in the midline (Fig. 9.11). The inside landmarks are 7 mm anterior to the posterior cruciate ligament and in the midline (Fig. 9.12).

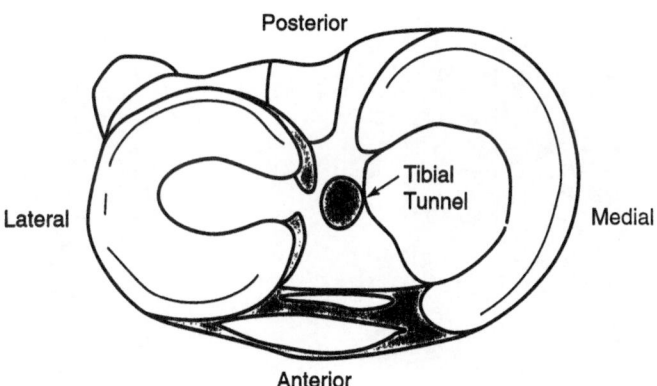

FIGURE 9.12. The landmarks for placement of the tibial guide wire.

Tunnel Malposition: Anterior Femoral Tunnel

Problem

The result of the anterior femoral tunnel placement is graft failure in flexion. The X-ray in Figure 9.13 shows the screw too anterior in the femur. This represents an anterior femoral tunnel. The graft will fail as the patient tries to regain flexion.

Often the graft is intact, but enlarged. Figure 9.14 shows an old anterior femoral tunnel, with the right arrow pointing out the new posterior tunnel. A second tunnel may be easily drilled behind this old tunnel.

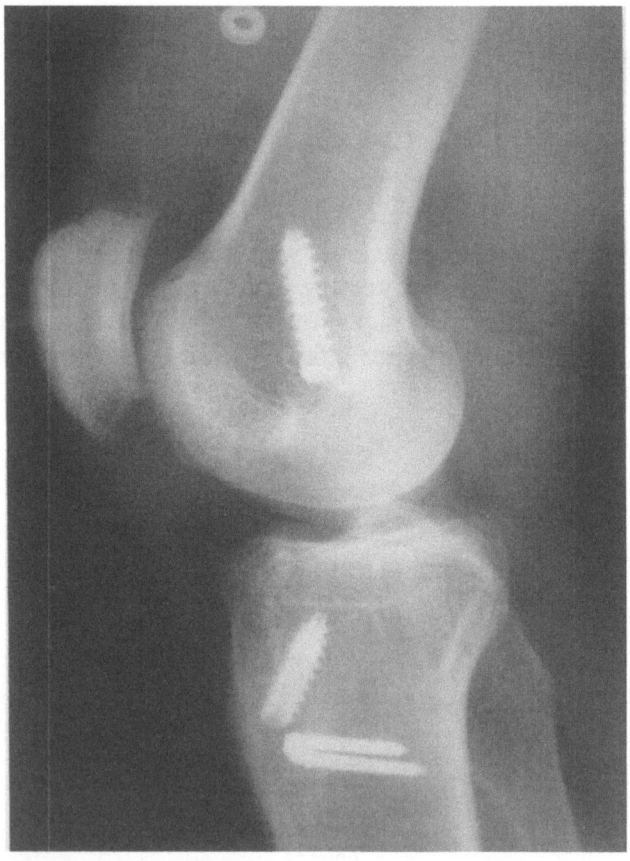

FIGURE 9.13. The X-ray of an anterior femoral tunnel.

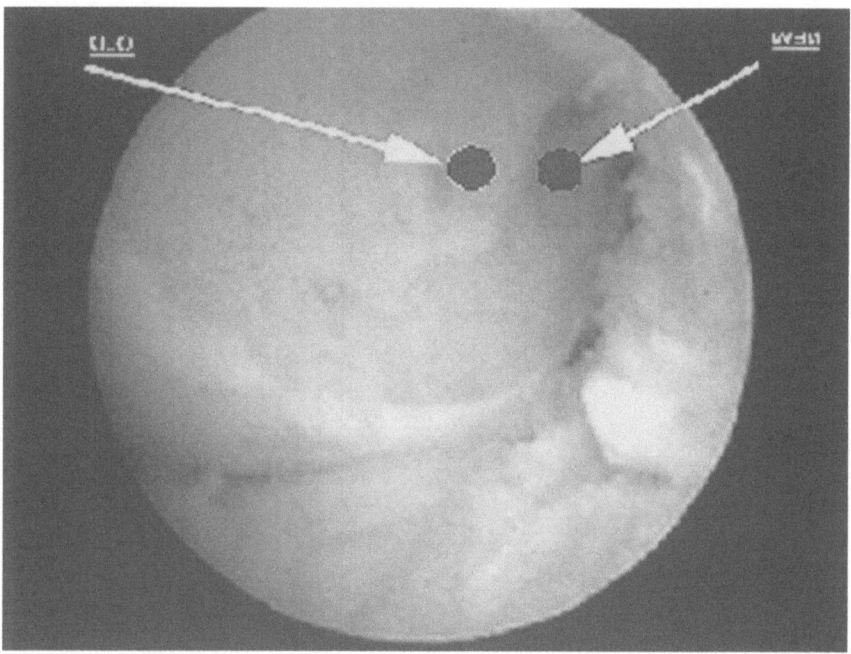

FIGURE 9.14. An old anterior femoral tunnel, with the right arrow pointing to the new posterior tunnel.

Solution

The most difficult situation is when the tunnel is only slightly anterior. The back of the condyle is rasped, and the graft is pulled into this over-the-top position and attached to the femur with staples or screw and washer. When the old tunnel is far anterior, another tunnel may be drilled behind. The second tunnel must be carefully inspected to be sure that it does not communicate with the anterior tunnel. If these tunnels are confluent, then the anterior tunnel may be filled with bone from the coring reamer or a BioScrew.

Prevention

Prevent the tunnel malposition in the femur by the use of the femoral aiming guide. This is inserted through the tibial tunnel with the knee flexed at 90°. The posterior fringe must be visualized. The guide wire is placed in the correct position and visualized before drilling. Figure 9.15 demonstrates the use of the Bullseye femoral aiming guide placed in the over-the-top position with the knee flexed at 90°. The size of the

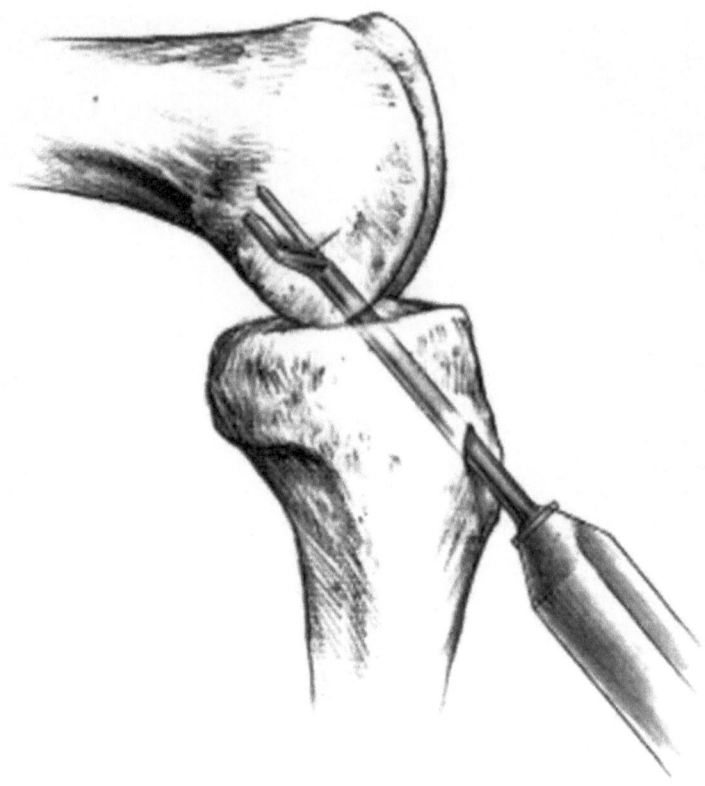

FIGURE 9.15. The femoral aiming device.

offset is determined by the size of the tunnel. For example a 7-mm offset is selected for a 10-mm tunnel.

Posterior Blowout of Femoral Tunnel

Problem

Figure 9.16 shows the thin posterior wall of the femoral tunnel, which indicates a weak posterior wall. The use of the interference screw would be contraindicated. It would not be strong enough to insert an interference screw. The screw would force the bone plug of the graft out the back of the tunnel, and loss of fixation would result.

Solution

When the back wall blowout is recognized, change from interference screw to Endo-button fixation. Another solution is to use the two-

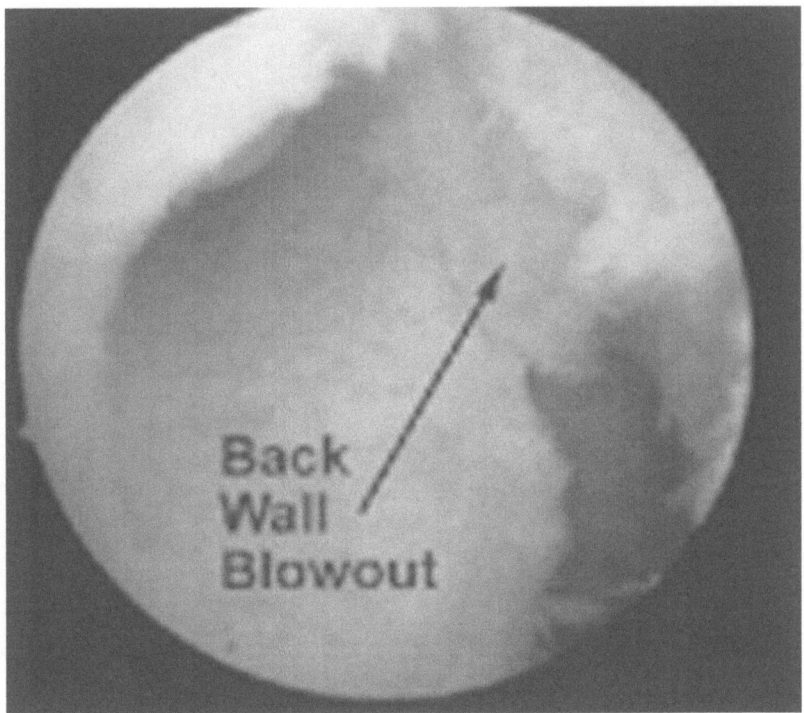

FIGURE 9.16. The back wall blowout.

incision technique, with the interference screw placed from outside in. It is also possible to advance the screw and graft farther up into the femoral tunnel. This is only possible when the blowout is more than a few millimeters.

Prevention

Prevent the blowout by flexing the knee to 90°. Visualize posterior fringe and use a push/pull drill to make an initial footprint. If this is not blowing out the posterior wall or is not too anterior, then the drill bit can be advanced 35 mm up into the femur. The footprint of the femoral tunnel position is made before committing to drilling the femoral tunnel (Fig. 9.17).

Overdrilling K-Wire

Problem

When the drill bit fails to progress, it may be that the bit is drilling into the wire (Fig. 9.18). To determine if this is the problem, pull the drill back, remove the K-wire, and insert a new one.

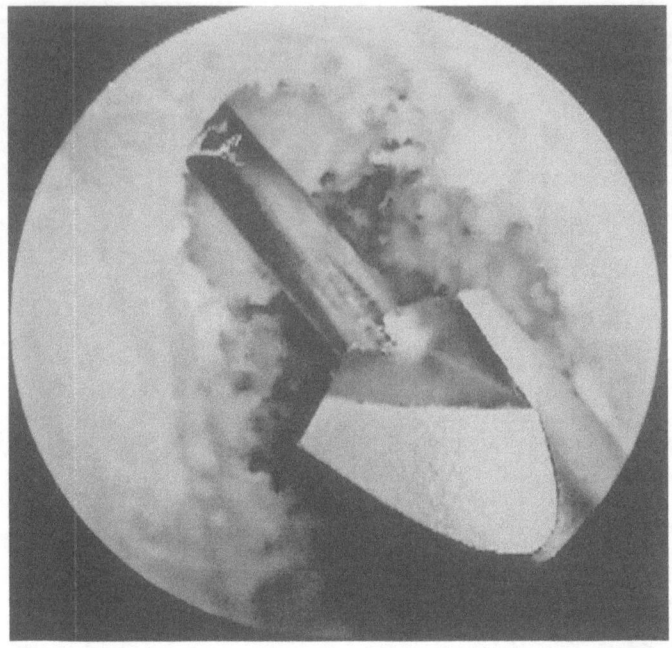

FIGURE 9.17. The footprint made by the drill bit.

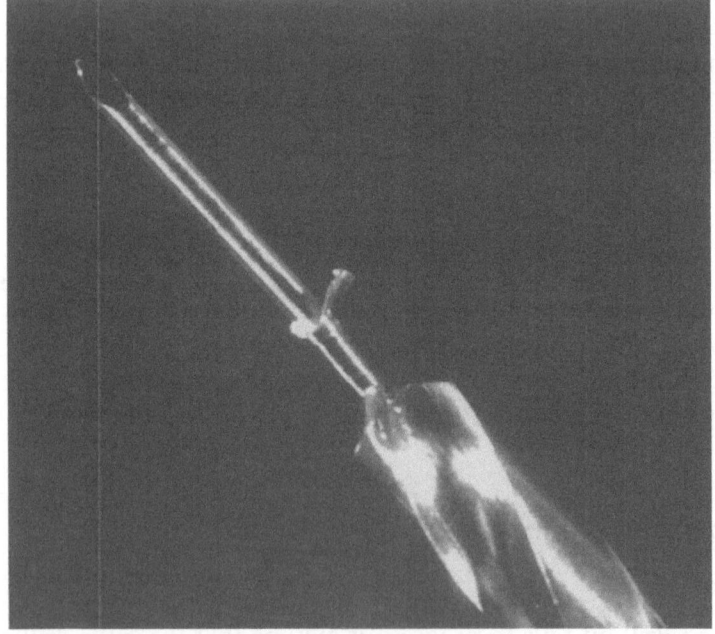

FIGURE 9.18. Cutting the K-wire with the drill bit.

Solution

The solution to the problem is to recognize it early and avoid completely drilling through the wire. If the wire is cut off in the middle of the tunnel, it is hard to retrieve.

Prevention

To prevent drilling the wire, watch the drill and piston over the wire to make sure that it is following the path of the wire. Do not be concerned about watching the monitor. Rather, watch the direction of the drill.

Piston Drilling to Follow the K-Wire: Lack of Visualization—The "Red Out"

Problem

Figure 9.19 is a typical picture of the red out. The surgeon should clear this before proceeding to operate. Do not run motorized devices in a red out.

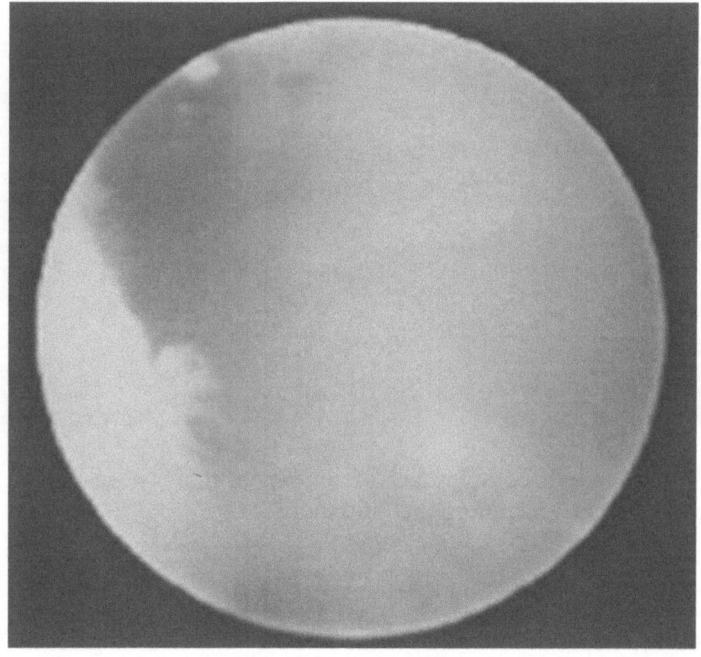

FIGURE 9.19. The red out.

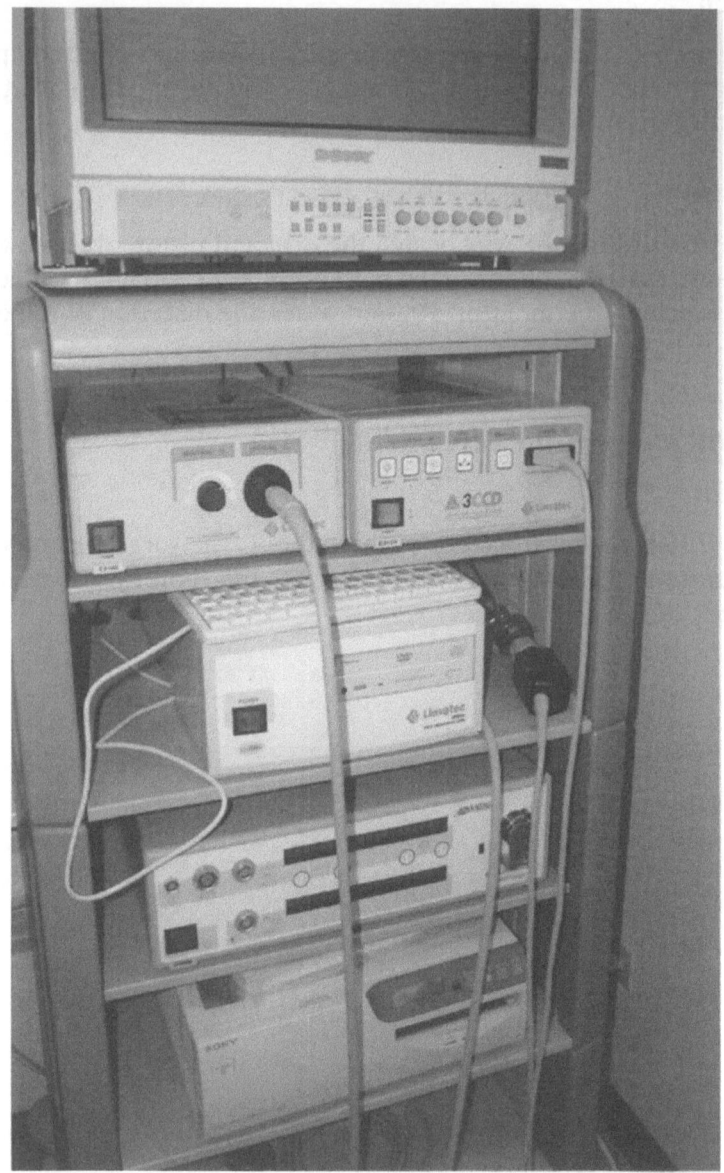

FIGURE 9.20. The arthroscopic stack of equipment that is necessary to perform arthroscopic surgery, including the fluid pump.

Solution

The remedy for the lack of visualization is the following:

- Increase the flow of the pump (Fig 9.20).
- Use one amp of Adrenalin in the saline.

- Inflate the tourniquet.
- Use suction to clear the joint and then reinfuse clear water.
- Use cautery to control the bleeders.

Loss of Fixation: Bone Plug Cut Off the Graft

Problem

The screw may cut the tendon off the bone plug if the screw does not follow the direction of the tunnel (Fig. 9.21).

Solution

The solution is to reverse direction of the graft. Put the tibial bone plug in femoral tunnel and fix this with an interference screw. On the other end, use a Krackow suture in the cut tendon end and tie over a button on the tibia (Fig. 9.2). A BioScrew may be used in the tunnel to help secure the graft. The sutures are placed in the tendon end of the graft and tied over a button or post.

Prevention

To prevent the screw from damaging the graft, visualize the angle of the screw during insertion. The screw should be parallel to the graft and convergent in the femoral tunnel (Fig. 9.22). It also helps to make a low anteromedial portal to insert the screw straight up the tunnel.

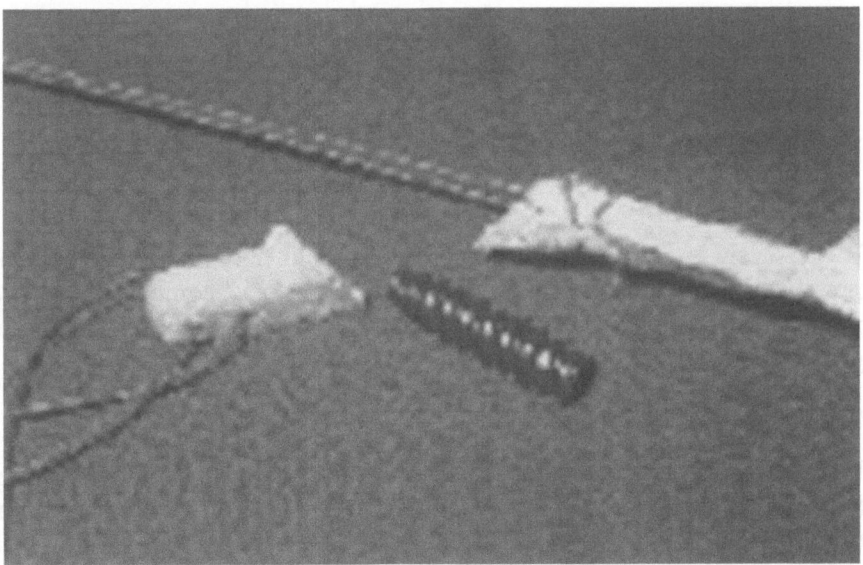

FIGURE 9.21. Cutting the graft with the screw.

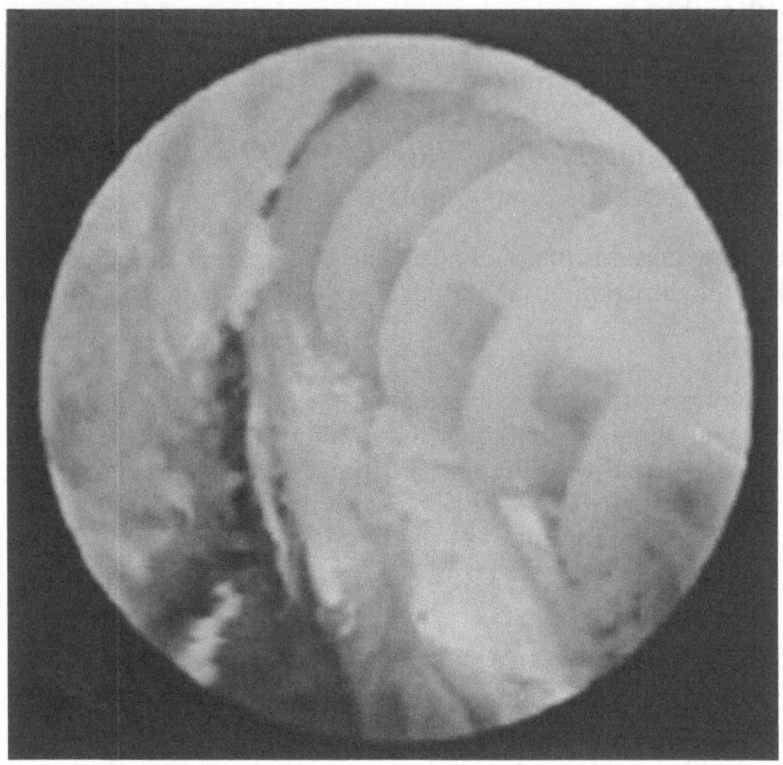

FIGURE 9.22. The insertion of the BioScrew into the femoral tunnel, parallel to the graft.

Loose Fixation of Interference Screws

Problem

If the screw is not put parallel to the tunnel, it may result in posterior penetration of the femoral tunnel. The screw may come loose in the joint. The appropriate size of screw, one that gives good purchase on the graft, must be used.

Solution

Use a two-pin passer to place the femoral screw in the femoral tunnel (Fig. 6.62). Visualize the screw guide wire in the notch for the tibial tunnel. If the guide wire is in the tunnel, the screw should follow the guide wire.

Prevention

In soft tissue graft fixation, use a screw that is the same size in the femoral tunnel and one size larger in the tibial tunnel. With the patellar tendon graft, measure the space between the bone plug and the sizing cylinder. If the space is less than 2mm, use a 7-mm screw. If the space is greater than 2mm, use a larger screw.

Graft Passage

Problem

If the graft is too tight in the tunnel, the leader sutures will break.

Solution

The solution is to remove the graft and dilate the tunnels up 1mm. The graft is resutured, lubricated, and passed.

Prevention

The prevention of a difficult graft passage is to make the patella bone plug 9mm so that it passes in a 10-mm tunnel. Size the soft tissue grafts to the same size as the tunnel. Do not soak the graft too long in saline, or it will swell. Measure the graft size after the suturing to make sure that it will pass easily.

Graft Tunnel Mismatch

Problem

The problem is that the bone plug sticks out of the tibia. It is impossible to use an interference fit screw in the tibial tunnel (Fig. 9.23).

Solution

The best solution is to trough the tibia and staple the tibial bone plug into the groove.

Prevention

Measuring graft and tunnel length can prevent this complication. The maximum length of the graft should be 9 to 10mm. If the patella tendon graft is 13mm, the bone plug may have to be flipped. Alan Barber has published the technique of flipping the bone plug back on the tendon graft and holding it with cerclage sutures.

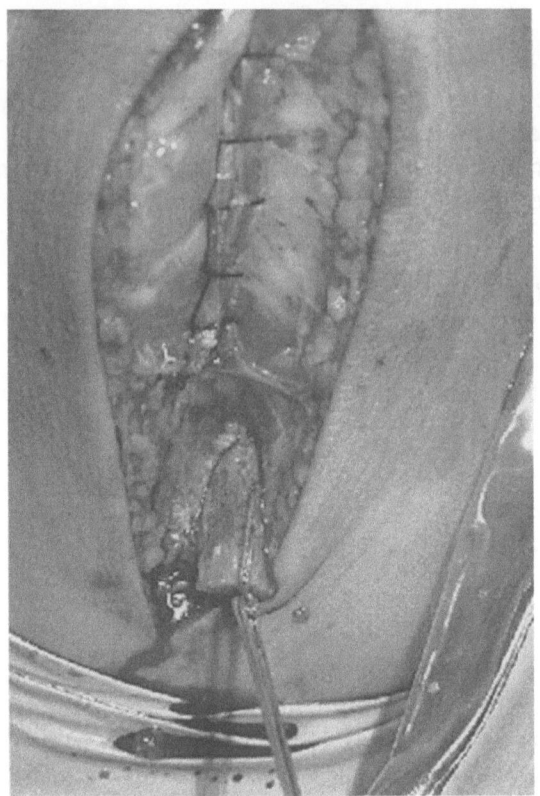

FIGURE 9.23. Graft tunnel mismatch.

Screw Divergence

Problem

A screw that is placed with a greater than 15° divergence results in loss of fixation. The screw appears to be normal from the anterior notch view, but on the posterior view of the sawbones model the screw has cut through the graft, and exited posteriorly (Fig. 9.24). This example is not only divergent, but has cut the bone plug off the graft.

Solution

The solution is to recognize the problem early and change the screw angle direction. It also helps to flex the knee 20° more than the tunnel angle.

Prevention

To prevent divergent screws, use a screw guide wire in the tunnel.

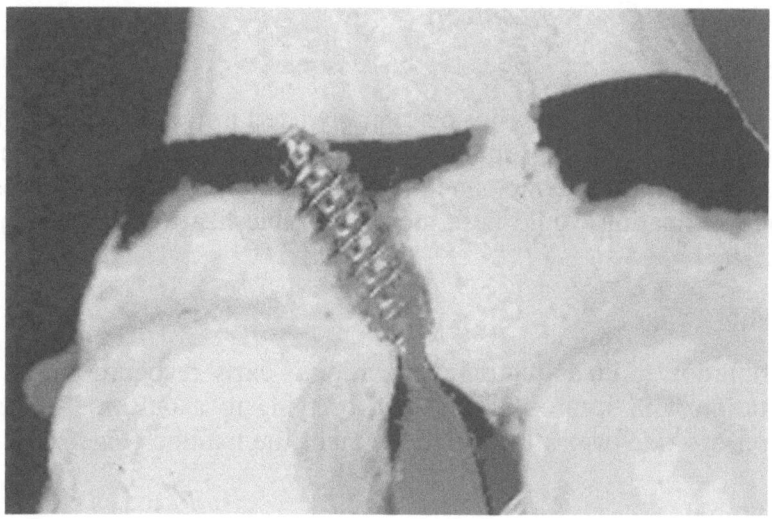

FIGURE 9.24. The screw protruding out the posterior aspect of the femoral tunnel.

Postoperative Complications

Late Patella Fracture

Problem

Figure 5.2 shows the transverse patella fracture that occurred three months postoperatively, with minor trauma.

Solution

The obvious solution is prompt open reduction and internal fixation (Fig. 5.3).

Prevention

The prevention of this complication is to avoid transverse saw cut overruns. An overrun of 2 mm may result in a fracture. If there are overruns, a burr may round off the corner and prevent a stress riser. The patella bone plug should be made boat shaped.

The transverse overruns that may result in stress risers (Fig. 5.4). To avoid these, cut the end of the patellar plug in a boat shape (Fig. 5.5).

Inadequate Graft Fixation

Problem

The soft tissue graft may not be securely fixed if there is reduced bone density. This can be a problem with the hamstring graft slipping under a BioScrew in osteopenic bone (Fig. 9.25). In this situation, a cross-pin or button fixation would be a more favorable fixation on the femoral side.

Solution

The solution to inadequate graft fixation is early recognition and augmentation with sutures over a post or tying to a button. The leader sutures are tied over a button to augment the fixation (Fig. 6.68).

Prevention

The prevention of weak fixation is to pick a fixation that is appropriate for the individual. The activities of daily living require at least 400N strength of the devices. Therefore, these fixation devices must exceed the 400N. Table 9.1 and Table 9.2 summarize the strength of fixation devices.

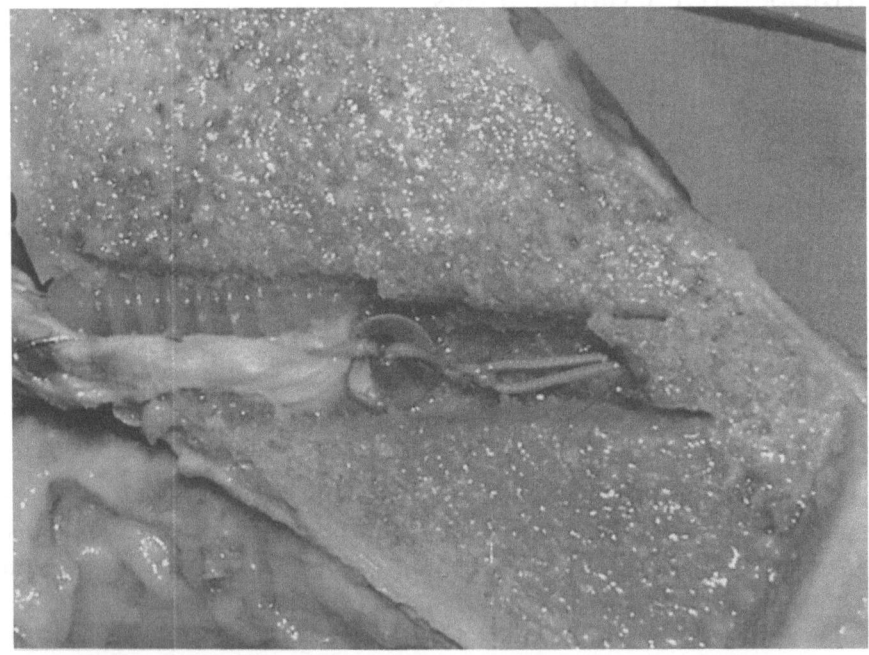

FIGURE 9.25. Interference screw fixation is bone-quality dependent.

TABLE 9.1. Femoral fixation devices: Pullout strength (load to failure).

Closed loop endobutton	1300N
Arthrex cross pin	1000N
Bone mulch screw	1000N
Mitek cross pin fixation	1000N
BioScrew and Endopearl	800N
Endo-button and tape	500N
BioScrew alone	400N
Mitek anchor	600N

Global Stiffness or Arthrofibrosis

Problem

The treatment of arthrofibrosis or global stiffness is very frustrating for the patient, therapist and surgeon (Fig. 9.26). Global arthrofibrosis is likely an inflammatory disease of unknown etiology. This is a very difficult clinical situation to treat.

Solution

The solution is early aggressive conservative treatment with appropriate pain management. Make sure that there is not an element of reflex sympathetic dystrophy.

Prevention

Time the operation to avoid acute postinjury situation. Allow the tissues to heal and wait for full range of motion and reduction in the swelling. Follow an accelerated rehabilitation program that emphasizes early extension and weight bearing. Be aggressive with pain management. Use the CPM, Cryo-Cuff, intra-articular injection of morphine and bupivacaine, and the preemptive femoral nerve block.

TABLE 9.2. Tibial fixation devices: Pullout strength (load to failure).

Washer Loc	1000N
Screw and washer	900N
Intrafix	900N
Suture post	600N
BioScrew	400N
Two staples	500N
Button	300N
RCI screw	250N
Single staple	200N

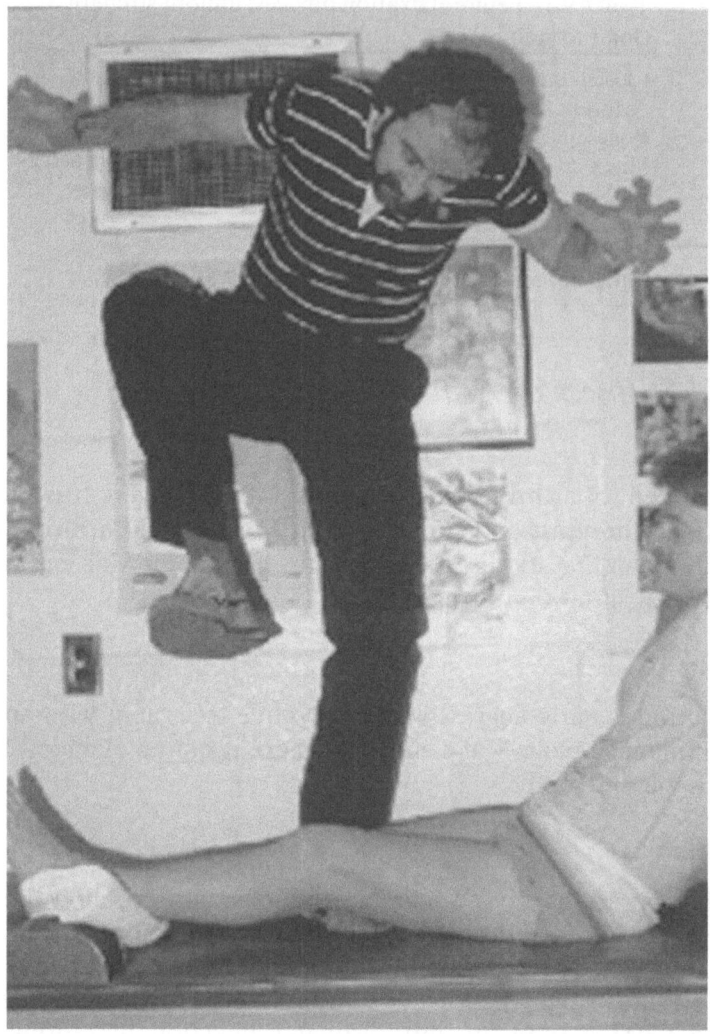

FIGURE 9.26. A crude method of regaining knee extension.

Loss of Flexion or Extension

Problem

The loss of flexion is due to suprapatellar pouch adhesions, or the tight patellofemoral joint. The loss of extension is the result of anterior notch scarring.

Solution

Extension

The solution for extension loss is to mobilize early with passive extension. If this fails, then arthroscopic excision of the scar and cyclops lesion.

Flexion

The solution to loss of flexion is to manually mobilize patella longitudinally. If this fails, then arthroscopic medial/lateral retinacular release should be done. The patella is mobilized by the therapist to regain the mobility of the patellofemoral joint (Fig. 8.6).

Prevention

Extension

The prevention of loss of extension is to emphasize early extension exercises. Use the CPM in full extension. Maintain the use of the extension splint and early full weight bearing. The early aggressive extension exercise with the use of a heel raise (Fig. 8.1).

Flexion

The prevention of flexion loss is early passive flexion with wall slides. The exercise bike should be used with no tension. The use of wall slides to encourage early flexion (Fig. 8.2).

Recurrent Instability

Problem

The problem of recurrent instability or failure of the reconstruction has several causes. Reinjury is one of the common causes of failure. The most common cause of failure is incorrect placement of the tunnels, especially the femoral tunnel. Loss of fixation, especially anterior placement of the femoral tunnel, is the common cause of graft elongation by flexion. The final unusual cause of failure is biological lack of graft incorporation.

Solution

Be thorough in attempting to identify cause of laxity by plain X-rays and MRI. Surgically correct the error, if indicated.

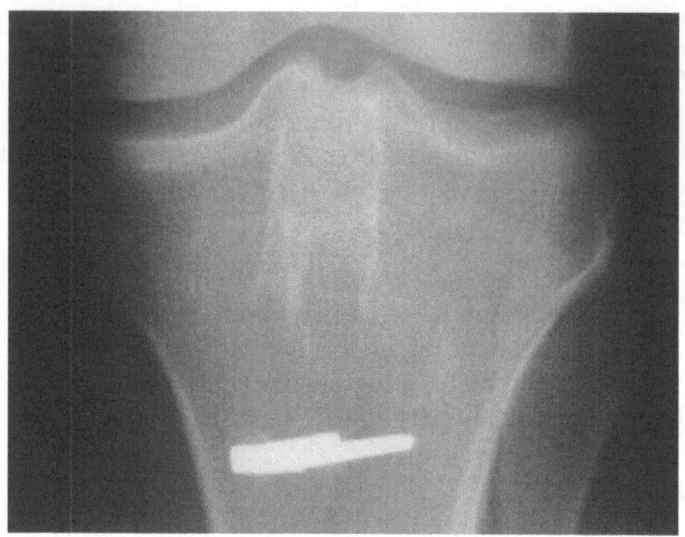

FIGURE 9.27. Tibial tunnel expansion.

Prevention

Splint or use a functional brace for six weeks postoperatively to prevent reinjury because of slip and fall. Use adequate soft tissue fixation in osteopenic bone. Back off physiotherapy, if early laxity detected. Use X-ray to confirm tunnel and screw position postoperatively.

Problem

Tunnel expansion after ACL reconstruction (Fig. 9.27).

Solution

This does not seem to have any clinical significance in short-term follow-up, and thus no treatment is necessary. This may become a problem at revision surgery, and very large tunnels may have to be bone grafted.

Prevention

It is felt that placing the fixation at the aperture of the tunnel would reduce the motion of the graft in the tunnel, reducing the radiological finding of tunnel enlargement.

10
Results

Pressman and Johnson have reviewed the early results of ACL reconstruction with BioScrew fixation of hamstring grafts in the following unpublished article, which is based on a presentation at AANA. This study prospectively evaluates a cohort of patients treated and followed for two years using a Poly-L-lactic acid screw (BioScrew).

Methods

A prospective study was undertaken to assess the effectiveness of the double-looped semitendinosus and gracilis graft secured with a biodegradable interference fixation screw (BioScrew). To be included, a patient had to meet the following criteria: a complete ACL tear, knee instability as manifested by positive Lachman test and positive pivot-shift test, a KT-1000 manual maximum side-to-side difference of greater than 5mm, and a commitment to return for at least two years of follow-up. Patients were excluded if they had an active infection preoperatively or multiple coincident ligament injuries (PCL, MCL, LCL, posterolateral corner). Previous knee ligament reconstruction was not an exclusionary criterion, and several of the patients included had revision surgery.

Preoperative assessments included a history, physical examination and radiographs. Baseline KT measurements at 20lbs, 30lbs, and maximum manual side-to-side difference were obtained. The surgical findings and procedures performed were recorded.

All patients underwent the same procedure: an arthroscope-assisted ACL reconstruction using a double-looped semitendinosus and gracilis autograft from the ipsilateral limb. The graft was secured at the proximal and distal sites with a BioScrew, and fixation was periodically supplemented on the tibial side with a periosteal button (Ethicon, J&J, Boston, MA).

Postoperative assessment included the IKDC score, KT tests, examination, and radiographs. The BioScrews are composed of purified poly

L-Lactide (containing 45% crystalline polymer). These screws were available in 7, 8, and 9 mm sizes for the tibia and femur. A 25-mm long screw was used in each case. These screws are cannulated and are placed over a Nitinol guide wire to prevent divergent placement of the screw.

Surgical Technique

The semitendinosus and gracilis tendons are harvested through an oblique anterior-medial incision along the upper border of the pes-anserine tendons. Turning down of the medial corner of the pes anserinus identified the tendons. Both were harvested with a closed-looped tendon stripper. The tendons, which ranged in length from 20 cm to 24 cm, were covered with a moist sponge for later preparation.

Any meniscal and interarticular pathology was then addressed, and the grafts were prepared (Fig. 6.43). The best 19 cm of each graft was trimmed from the tendons, and the proximal end of one was sewn to the distal end of the other with No. 2 Ti-Cron suture. The tendon was then looped over a No. 5 Ti-Cron suture to be used to pull the graft into the knee. The proximal 3 cm of the tendon, which would reside in the femoral tunnel, was then sewn to bundle each of the four strands together for the portion with No. 0 Vicryl suture. The proximal and distal ends of the graft were then sized with cylindrical sizing tubes at 0.5 mm increments.

A soft tissue notchplasty was performed and only if bony impingement was noted was a bony notchplasty performed. Using the Howell Tibial Guide (ArthroCare, Biomet, Warsaw, IN), a guide wire was introduced into the tibia at an angle of approximately 50° to 55°, a tibial tunnel of approximately 5 cm in length was created. The position of the guide wire was verified with the arthroscope.

A tibial drill of the corresponding size to the graft was introduced into the tibia to create a tibial tunnel. A transtibial guide was selected to leave a 1-mm to 2-mm posterior bone bridge. The guide was placed and was followed by placement of a guide wire. After the verification of the location of a mark made on the femur by the drill to indicate the location of the femoral tunnel, a femoral tunnel was drilled to 30 mm.

The tibial aperture was cleaned and the femoral tunnel compacted with a notcher. The knee was then cycled and the femoral fixation tested. A femoral BioScrew guide wire was then introduced ensuring that the screw and wire were placed parallel with the graft. The femoral BioScrew was then introduced into the femoral tunnel.

With the arthroscope in the joint, a guide wire was then passed into the joint anterior to the graft through the tibial tunnel. The knee was then placed at 20° of extension on the table. With distal tension on the graft and a posterior force was applied to the tibia, the tibial BioScrew was introduced. No specific effort was made to place the BioScrew at the aperture of the tibial tunnel. Secondary fixation was used on the tibia in 15 cases where the bony fixation of the tibial screw seemed suboptimal intraoperatively.

BioScrew sizes were selected such that the femoral screw was of the same size or 1 mm smaller than the tunnel drilled and the tibial screw was generally 1 mm larger in diameter than the tibial tunnel drill bit.

Results

During the period of evaluation from December 1997 to April 1998, a total of 174 knees underwent ACL reconstruction using this technique. Complete two-year follow-up (mean 2.4 years) including IKDC forms and KT results are available for 49 patients. These data represent preliminary results on these patients for the BioScrew.

The average age of the patients in this study was 33.1 +/- 7.0 years (range 16 to 49). All patients had chronic ACL tears at the time of operation (more than three months after injury). Four patients had failed a previous ACL reconstruction, and two patients had undergone remote primary repair of their ACL. There were 37 males (76%) and 12 females (24%). Twenty-one right and twenty-eight left knees were affected. Associated surgical findings included chondromalacia, meniscal tears, and loose bodies. A medial partial medial meniscectomy of less than one-third was performed in 21 cases (41%), a complete medial meniscectomy in 2 (4%), a partial lateral meniscectomy of less than one-third in 18 (36%), and a complete lateral meniscectomy in 1 (2%).

Follow-up KT tests showed an average laxity with a maximum manual force of 1.5 mm ± 3.6 mm at one year and 1.25 mm ± 2.82 mm at two years. Patients were further divided into categories of laxity with 33 (67%) patients having 0 mm to 2 mm of laxity; 13 patients (27%) having 3 mm to 5 mm of laxity, and 2 (4.1%) having greater than 5 mm of laxity. One patient in the greater than 5 mm laxity group and 3 patients in the 3 mm to 5 mm laxity group represented revision surgical procedures.

At final follow-up, one patient had a persistent effusion, one patient lacked 5° of extension, and four patients lacked 5° of flexion.

The Lachman test was normal in 32 patients, grade 1+ in 12 patients, and grade 3+ in two patients. One patient was felt to have mild PCL instability, and two patients had mild posterolateral instability on emergency room testing at 30°. At the final follow-up, four patients had a 1+ pivot glide, and one had a 3+ pivot shift. No instances of Bio-Screw breakage occurred.

Radiographs were taken of the knees at the two-year follow-up visit to complete the IKDC forms.

Tunnels were measured at their widest point, at the aperture, the midpoint, and 1 cm from the distal aspect of the tunnel. In 36 of the 49 cases (73%), the X-rays were available for secondary review of the tunnels. The morphology of the tunnel, the width of its widest point, the width of the aperture, and the cross-sectional area were measured and compared to mechanical outcome.

Significant tunnel expansion (Group C) was identified in 10 cases (28%). In these cases, the tibial tunnel was expanded in seven, and femoral tunnel expansion was identified in seven cases. In six cases, the expansion could be considered to be significant, with the widest point of both tunnels measuring 15 mm. Four of the ten cases in group C had between 3 mm and 5 mm of laxity at maximum manual force at the two-year follow-up mark. No significant correlations existed by comparison with the Spearman correlation coefficient between final IKDC score or KT-score or with the measurements of the tunnels at the aperture, midsection, widest point, or most distant part of the tunnel. In the five cases where both tunnels measured greater than 15 mm, on at least one radiograph, two cases were in the 3 mm to 5 mm group.

From the other perspective, 18 cases with available radiographs at two-years had less than 2 mm of laxity, seven had 3 mm to 5 mm of laxity, and one had greater than 5 mm of laxity on a maximum manual force KT examination. In four of the seven cases, the morphology of the tunnel could be classified as expansive as opposed to cylindrical and filling in with bone (57%). However in 6 of the 18 cases (33%) with less than 2 mm of laxity, similarly expansive tunnels were identified. The extent of aperture widening did not correlate with clinical laxity or IKDC score at two-year follow-up.

Multiple statistical comparisons were made to identify positive predictive factors, which resulted in an increased trend for a patient to fall into the 3 mm to 5 mm laxity group at two years. Specifically using post hoc ANOVA, ANCOVA comparisons, Spearman rank correlations, and unpaired two-tailed student t-tests, it was concluded that gender, patient age, the use of secondary tibial fixation, and the magnitude of preoperative instability and laxity could not be associated with an increased KT manual maximum laxity or an increased prevalence of patients in the 3 mm to 5 mm laxity group. Comparisons were repeated after the exclusion of the revision surgical procedures, but this did not affect the results.

TABLE 10.1. The correlation of IKDC scores and gender, use of the secondary tibial button fixation and revision.

	Total	Male	Female	Tibial button	Revision
IKDC	84.5 ± 15.3	85.6 ± 16.0	81.6 ± 13	79.3 ± 19.8	74.0 ± 5.0
KT side to side (2 yr)	1.25 ± 2.89	1.53 ± 2.25	1.67 ± 2.35*	1.00 ± 3.60	5.00 ± 2.00

The IKDC activity score represents a composite score of subjective questionnaires and clinical function. Activity in sedentary activities (activities of daily living), light activities (nonpivotal sports), moderate activities (tennis, skiing), and strenuous activity (jumping, pivoting sports) were graded by the patients. These subjective scores are combined with a mathematical formula to create the IKDC score. These scores were calculated at two years to be 84.5 ± 15.3 (Table 10.1). Age, gender, and meniscal pathology were not associated with a significant change in the IKDC score (Table 10.1 and Table 10.2). Patients with greater than 5 mm laxity were associated with a significantly decreased IKDC score from those with 0 mm to 2 mm or 3 mm to 5 mm ($p > 0.02$). There was also a trend toward a decreased score in patients with radiographic evidence of degenerative changes ($p < 0.21$).

Where BioScrew fixation was used in the case of a revision ACL in four cases, a 3 mm to 5 mm side-to-side difference was obtained in 3 cases, and a greater than 5 mm laxity was obtained in 1 case. Thus, in no case was an optimal mechanical result (<2 mm) achieved. The significantly increased laxity ($p < 0.005$) in revision cases was also associated with a trend toward a decreased IKDC score with it averaging 74 in this group ($p < 0.17$).

Discussion

There has been a trend among some investigators to shift to an increased reliance on the semitendinosus graft for ACL reconstruction. This has been promoted by multiple studies, which favor its use after

TABLE 10.2. The IKDC scores comparing meniscectomy and degenerative X-ray changes.

	Total	Lateral meniscectomy	Medial meniscectomy	Degenerative OA on X-ray
IKDC	84.5 ± 15.3	88.9 ± 11.3	33.9 ± 33.4	77.9 ± 16.1
KT side to side (2 yr)	1.25 ± 2.89	1.23 ± 1.91	1.50 ± 2.56	1.29 ± 1.89

consideration of donor site morbidity and rehabilitation without the sacrifice of functional outcome.

This study served to evaluate the use of the BioScrew for hamstring ACL reconstruction. The screw is made of poly-L-lactide and biodegrades over several years. It has been shown to work well in patellar tendon graft ACL reconstructions. The adaptation of this interference screw technique to this graft has several advantages, including its straightforward technique, the avoidance of graft cutting (previously seen with metal screws), and ultimate resorption of the graft. An additional advantage is that these screws are cannulated, allowing accurate placement of the screws into the appropriate tunnels.

These results demonstrate excellent clinical results in terms of patient satisfaction and outcome. The average IKDC score was 84.6 +/− 15.3, and the maximum manual KT-2000 side-to-side difference was 1.25 mm at two years. The results indicated that 33 patients (67%) had 0 mm to 2 mm of laxity; 13 patients (27%) had 3 mm to 5 mm of laxity, and 2 patients (4.1%) had greater than 5 mm of laxity. One of the two patients with greater than 5 mm of laxity was satisfied with the stability of the knee and reported an IKDC of 93; the other represented a clinical and mechanical failure of the graft. These results are consistent with other series, which have reported on soft tissue fixation of hamstring grafts with the Endo-button Acufex (Smith-Nephew Richards, Warsaw, IN).

The results of this technique in revision ACL surgery were suboptimal, with increased mechanical laxity existing in each case. While this may result from either the effects on the multiply operated limb or increased laxity of associated structures, efforts should focus on improvements in these results. Intraoperative attention should focus on ensuring that when screw fixation is used, the revision tunnels do not communicate with existing tunnels forming an oval tunnel with insufficient strength to support the screw-tendon fixation.

An internal evaluation of the cohort of patients treated at the same sports medicine facility revealed that there was an increased prevalence of patients with between 3 mm and 5 mm of laxity on maximum manual KT-2000 measurements at two years (7.1% BPTB vs 27% ST), when comparing patients treated with the patellar tendon graft to those treated with a four-bundle hamstring graft using bioabsorbable screw fixation. Although this degree of laxity is consistent with other published series using soft tissue fixation of hamstring grafts, our group wished to closely evaluate these results.

A three-month review of patients treated with BioScrew presented at the AANA in 1999 suggested an increased laxity in female patients. These results were not supported by a review of the first 49 patients of this cohort to undergo a two-year follow-up (figure age and gender, etc.). Similarly, no correlation between gender, age, preoperative laxity, the presence of meniscal pathology, and the use of secondary tibial fixation in the form of a polypropylene button was identified. Other studies have also been unable to show a gender bias to poorer outcome.

Statistical tests were composed of ANOVA and ANCOVA analyses of variance to determine the effects of these factors on the side-to-side difference manual-maximum KT-2000 scores and the IKDC scores, which were used as outcome measures at two-year follow-up. Additional tests with Spearman's rank correlation were used to identify the correlations between the size of the graft (bone tunnels drilled) and the size differential between the drilled tunnel and the screw size and measurements of tunnel dilation. Again, no specific correlation was identified.

An evaluation of the radiographic morphology of the tunnels was performed. While osteolytic areas up to 1 cm in diameter have been accompanied by pure polyglycolide (PGA) screws between 6 and 12 weeks after implantation, these findings have been very rare with a pure poly-L-lactic acid screw such as the BioScrew. This polymer has a six-month half-life and degrades by hydrolysis, as shown by Barber. In other studies the use of this screw has not been associated with osteolysis.

Of 36 radiographs reviewed, it was not uncommon to see evidence of resorption of the screw adjacent to the femoral tunnel at the screw-femur interface. In ten cases the tunnels were expansive, having a diameter measurement on at least one radiograph, of greater than 15 mm. In six of these cases, both the tibial and femoral tunnels measured greater than 15 mm on at least one view. In only four of these ten cases was this expansive tunnel with a radiographic diameter of 15 mm on at least one radiograph associated with a KT-2000 side-to-side value of greater than 3 mm.

While this appearance of the poly-L-lactic acid screws has not previously been reported, it did not affect the outcome measures. The presence of tunnel expansion could represent graft motion or an osseous response to screw resorption. At the time of these procedures, attention was not attuned to aperture fixation to prevent graft motion at the graft-joint interface.

To minimize the radiographic evidence of graft motion at the apertures of the bone tunnels and to decrease the occurrence of patients with 3 mm to 5 mm of laxity at two years, our group has made several changes to the BioScrew technique from that used in this cohort. A construct with an Endopearl is now established so that a 25-mm femoral BioScrew opposes the Endopearl at the femoral cortical aperture. This enables the advantage of the femoral cortical bite with the screw, the benefit of the Endopearl, and aperture femoral fixation. The proximal

3 cm of the graft is now sutured with No. 2 Ti-Cron to improve the screw-graft fixation (Pinczewski, personal communication).

On the tibial side, the BioScrew is advanced to the distal cortex. Secondary tibial fixation in terms of tying the graft over a button is now used in all cases. The femoral screw size used is now the same as the femoral tunnel, and the tibial screw is 1 mm larger than the tibial tunnel size. The tibia is drilled two sizes smaller than the measured graft size and cannulated tunnel dilators are used to compact the bone of the bone tunnels.

In conclusion, the BioScrew is a safe and effective means of securing a soft four-bundle hamstring graft. Inferior mechanical results are obtained using this technique alone in revision ACL surgery. Recent changes to technique have been directed at the identification of improvements in graft fixation strength and aperture fixation to further improve results.

The Controversies

Timing of the Operation

Most surgeons will delay the operation until the pain and swelling have decreased and the range of motion of the knee has improved. There is no definite time frame to achieve this. Some patients are ready in one week, and others take six weeks. If there is a loss of extension, then imaging must be done to determine if this is the stump of the ligament or a displaced bucket-handle meniscal tear. The meniscal tear should be reduced and repaired early. The knee is then rehabilitated to regain the range of motion, and the ACL reconstruction can be carried out at a second stage.

Patient Selection

The operative procedure should be done on a compliant patient. The abnormally lax patient will present problems in achieving stability.

The Type of Graft: Patellar Tendon vs. Semitendinosus

The conventional wisdom is that the young pivoting contact sport athlete should have a patellar tendon reconstruction. Patients with pre-existing patellofemoral symptoms or who are only involved in recreational activities should undergo a semitendinosus reconstruction. The metaanalysis of the five studies in the literature that compare the hamstrings and the patellar tendon grafts concluded that the outcome is virtually the same for the two procedures. The only significant difference is that with the patellar tendon graft there is a 20% greater chance of returning to the same level of preinjury sports participation.

Notchplasty

The current trend is to do less notchplasty. The notch only has to be large enough to accommodate the graft. In most cases only the soft tissue needs to be removed to visualize the over the top position.

Pretensioning of the Graft, Especially the Semitendinosus

This has become less of an issue since we have moved to the interference screw fixation of the semitendinosus. The fixation is near the tunnel entrance and reduces the bungee effect of periosteal fixation.

Tensioning of the Graft

The graft should be tensioned with about 10 lb to 15 lb of tension at 20° of knee flexion. This is the position of the least tension in the native ACL.

Fixation: BioScrew

The fixation of grafts with the bioabsorbable screw is evolving into the preferred method of fixation. The blunt metal screw has become the standard, and the bioabsorbable screw has advantages over the metal screw, so it should become the standard of the future.

Timing of Return to Sport

The most important advance in ACL reconstruction in the past decade has been the concept of accelerated rehabilitation as proposed by Shelbourne. This has reduced the problems of limited range of motion and patellofemoral pain and has increased the return to sports participation. It has also reduced the time of return to sports from 12 months to 4 months.

Recently, the popular press has discussed athletes who return to sports in six to eight weeks. In the author's opinion, the athlete may be rehabilitated, but has the biology of soft tissue healing had a chance to incorporate the graft? Most surgeons feel that it takes four to six months for the athlete to recover after autogenous ACL graft reconstruction.

Use of a Brace

The use of a functional brace after ACL reconstruction is still a debatable issue. The author feels that if a patient undergoes a reconstruction, a brace is not necessary for return to sport. If the patient elects to undergo conservative treatment, the functional brace is a mainstay of that treatment.

Conclusions

The patellar tendon is a reliable graft that allows the athlete to resume sports early. The procedure has significant postoperative patellofemoral pain and stiffness. This may be reduced with aggressive rehabilitation to regain extension and to mobilize the patella.

The semitendinosus graft is the up-and-coming graft choice. The advantages are less harvest site morbidity. The disadvantages are the variable graft size and longer time to return to sports.

In summary, there are several graft choices. The decision must be made between patient and surgeon. The author is suggesting that the surgeon should have more than one option available to offer to the patient.

The more important issue in ACL reconstruction is not the graft choice, but is in placing the tunnels in the correct position (Fig. 10.1). There are several guides available for both the tibial and the femoral tunnels that help the surgeon place the guide wire in the proper position. At that time, if the surgeon is not sure of the positioning, then the fluoroscopy can be used to determine the correct position.

The assessment of the outcome of the treatment should be done by both subjective and objective functional outcome measurements. Several measurement scales are available, such as the International Knee Documentation Committee form or IKDC. When the outcome measurements are made on this scale, they can be interpreted by anyone. At the present time, only 43% of the members of the ACL study group use this form; most say that the form is not user friendly. We must continue to strive for a universal system that will make it easier to judge the success of different types of treatment of the ACL injured knee.

The Future

The current surgical technique of autogenous graft harvest, with tunnel preparation, will change very little. The changes will come in the evolution of graft fixation with bioabsorbable materials.

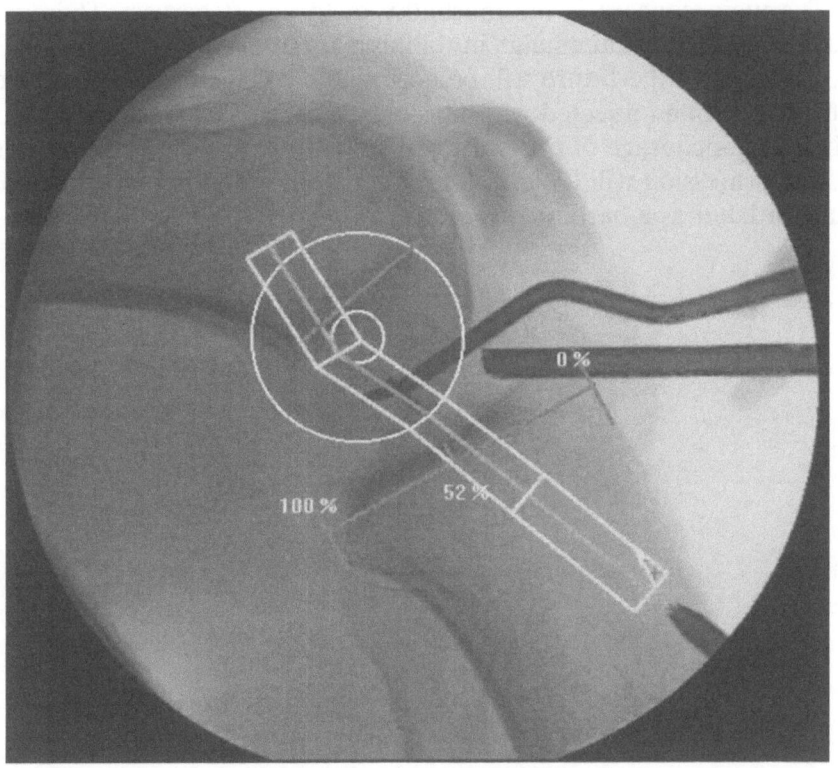

Graft

	Length	Diameter
Proximal	25 mm	11 mm
Distal	30 mm	11 mm
Tendon	45 mm	
Total	100 mm	

Graft-tunnel matching

Graft length	100 mm
Proximal length	25 mm
IAD	<u>20 mm</u>
Required length	55 mm
Actual length	58 mm
Inside tibia	30 mm
Outside tibia	0 mm

Distal Block

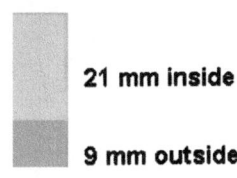

21 mm inside

9 mm outside

FIGURE 10.1. X-ray assisted placement of the femoral tunnel. (X-ray image courtesy of Burt Klos.)

The main concern is the morbidity of the graft harvest. There will have to be significant change in thinking about grafts.

The graft of the future will be a synthetic collagen scaffold selected off the shelf and injected with fibroblastic cells to produce collagen in vivo. The anchorage of this graft will be with bioabsorbable materials.

The profession will look back on the patellar tendon not as the gold standard, but as a barbaric procedure!

11
Readings

Aligetti P, Buzzi R, D'Andri S, Zaccherotti G. Patellofemoral problems after intraarticular anterior cruciate ligament reconstruction. Clin Orthop Related Res 1993;288:195–204.

Aligetti PB, Bazzi R, Zaccherotti G, De Biase P. Patellar tendon versus doubled semitendinosus and gracilis tendons for anterior cruciate ligament reconstruction. Am J Sports Med 1994;22(2):211–217.

Arendt E, Dick R. Knee injury patterns among men and women in collegiate basketball and soccer. NCAA data and review of literature. Am J Sports Med 1995;23(6):694–701.

Barber FA, et al. Preliminary results of an absorbable interference screw. Arthroscopy 1995;11:537–548.

Barber FA, Elrod BF, McGuire DA, Paulos LE. Is an anterior cruciate ligament reconstruction outcome age dependent? Arthroscopy 1996;12(6):720–725.

Barber FA, et al. Flipped patellar tendon autograft anterior cruciate ligament reconstruction. Arthroscopy 2000;16:483–490.

Barrett GR, Field LD. Comparison of patella tendon versus patella tendon/Kennedy ligament augmentation device for anterior cruciate ligament reconstruction: study of results, morbidity, and complications. Arthroscopy 1993;9(6):624–632.

Bartolozzi P, Salvi M, Velluti C. Long-term follow-up of 53 cases of chronic lesion of the anterior cruciate ligament treated with an artificial Dacron Stryker ligament. Ital J Orthop Traumatol 1990;16(4):467–480.

Brand J Jr, Weiler A, Caborn DN, Brown CH Jr, Johnson DL. Graft fixation in cruciate ligament reconstruction. Am J Sports Med 2000;28(5):761–774.

Brandsson S, et al. A comparison of results in middle-aged and young patients after anterior cruciate ligament reconstruction. Arthroscopy 2000;16:178–182.

Brown CH Jr, Steiner ME, Carson EW. The use of hamstring tendons for anterior cruciate ligament reconstruction. Technique and results. Clin Sports Med 1993;12:723–756.

Brown GC, Rosenberg TD, Deffner KT. Inside-out meniscal repair using zone-specific instruments. Am J Knee Surg 1996;9:144–150.

Buckley SL, Barrack RL, Alexander AH. The natural history of conservatively treated partial anterior cruciate ligament tears. Am J Sports Med 1989;17:221–225.

Cannon WD Jr, Morgan CD. Meniscal repair: Arthroscopic repair techniques. Instr Course Lect 1994;43:77–96.

Cooley VJ, Deffner TMS, Rosenberg TD. Quadrupled semitendinosus anterior cruciate ligament reconstruction: 5-year results in patients without meniscus loss. Arthroscopy 2000;17:795–800.

Daniel D, Principles of knee ligament surgery. In: Knee Ligaments: Structure, Function, Injury, and Repair, Akeson WHA, Daniel DM, and O'Connor JJ (eds.). New York: Raven Press; 1990.

DeLee JE, Curtis R. Anterior cruciate ligament insufficiency in children. Clin Orthop 1983;172:112–118.

Engstrom B, Wredmark T, Westblad P. Patellar tendon or Leeds-Keio graft in the surgical treatment of anterior cruciate ligament ruptures. Intermediate results. Clin Orthop 1993;295:190–197.

Ettlinger CF, Johnson RJ, Shealy JE. A method to help reduce the risk of serious knee sprains incurred in alpine skiing. Am J Sports Med 1995;23: 531–537.

Fetto JF, Marshall JL. The natural history and diagnosis of anterior cruciate ligament insufficiency. Clin Orthop 1980;147:29–38.

Fowler PJ. Semitendinosus tendon anterior cruciate ligament reconstruction with LAD augmentation. Orthopedics 1993;16(4):449–53.

Fruensgaard S, Johannsen HV. Incomplete ruptures of the anterior cruciate ligament. J Bone Joint Surg 1989;71B:526–530.

Fukubayashi T, Ikeda K. Follow-up study of Gore-Tex artificial ligament–special emphasis on tunnel osteolysis. J Long-Term Effects Med Implants 10(4):267–277.

Fulkerson JP, Langeland R. An alternative cruciate reconstruction graft: The central quadriceps tendon. Arthroscopy 1995;11:252–254.

Griffin LY, Agel J, Albohm M, et al. Noncontact anterior cruciate ligament injuries: risk factors and prevention strategies. J Am Acad Orthop Surg 2000;8:141–150.

Hamner DL, Brown CH, Steiner ME, et al. Hamstring tendon grafts for reconstruction of the anterior cruciate ligament: Biomechanical evaluation of the use of multiple strands and tensioning techniques. J Bone Joint Surg 1999;81: 549–557.

Harmon KG, Ireland ML. Gender differences in noncontact anterior cruciate ligament injuries. Clin Sports Med year 19:287–302.

Hay Groves E. Operation for the repair of the cruciate ligaments. Lancet 1917; 2:674–675.

Henning CE, et al. Arthroscopic meniscal repair using an exogenous fibrin clot. Clin Orthop 1990;252:64–72.

Hewitt TE, Lindenfeld TN, Riccobene JV, et al. The effect of neuromuscular training on the incidence of knee injuries in female athletes. Am J Sports Med 1999;27: 699–705.

Howell SM, Taylor MA. Failure of reconstruction of the anterior cruciate ligament due to impingement by the intercondylar roof. J Bone Joint Surg 1993;75:1044–1055.

Jackson DW, Corsetti J, Simon TM. Biologic incorporation of allograft anterior cruciate ligament replacements. Clin Orthop 1996;(324):126–133.

Johnson RJ, Eriksson E, Haggmark T, et al. Five- to ten-year follow-up evaluation after reconstruction of the anterior cruciate ligament. Clin Orthop 1984;183:122–140.

Karageanes SJ, Blackburn K, Vangelos ZA. The association of the menstrual cycle with the laxity of the anterior cruciate ligament in adolescent female athletes. Clin J Sport Med 2000;10(3):162–168.

Kurzweil PR, Friedman MF. Meniscus resection, repair, and replacement. Arthroscopy 2002;18:33–39.

Lipscomb AB, Johnston RK, Snyder RB, Warburton MJ, Gilbert PP. Evaluation of hamstring strength following use of semitendinosus and gracilis tendons to reconstruct the anterior cruciate ligament. Am J Sports Med 1982;10:340–342.

Marder RA, Raskind JR, Carroll M. Prospective evaluation of arthroscopically assisted anterior cruciate ligament reconstruction, patellar tendon vs semitendinosus and gracilus tendons. Am J Sports Med 1991;19(5):478–484.

Martinek VF, Friedrich NF. To brace or not to brace? How effective are knee braces in rehabilitation? Orthopaed 1999;28(6):565–570.

Marumo K, Kumagae Y, Tanaka T, et al. Long-term results of anterior cruciate ligament reconstruction using semitendinosus and gracilis tendons with Kennedy ligament augmentation device compared with patellar tendon autografts. J Long-Term Effects Med Implants 2000;10:251–265.

Noyes FR, Barber SD. Allograft reconstruction of the anterior and posterior cruciate ligaments: report of ten-year experience and results. Instr Course Lect 1993;42:381–396.

Noyes FR, Barber SD, Simon R. High tibial osteotomy and ligament reconstruction in varus angulated, anterior cruciate ligament-deficient knees. A two- to seven-year follow-up study. Am J Sports Med 1993;21(1):2–12.

Noyes FR, Barber SD, Manine RE. Bone-patellar ligament-bone and fascia lata allografts for reconstruction of the anterior cruciate ligament. J Bone Joint Surg 1990;72:1125–1136.

Noyes FR, Butler DL, Grood ES, Zernicke RF, Hefzy MS. Biomechanical analysis of human ligament grafts used in knee-ligament repairs and reconstruction. J Bone Joint Surg 1984;66(3):344–352.

Noyes FR, Mooar LA, Moorman CT III, McGinniss GH. Partial tears of the anterior cruciate ligament. Progression to complete ligament deficiency. J Bone Joint Surg 1989;71(5):825–833.

Noyes FR, Mooar PA, Matthews DS, Butler DL. The symptomatic anterior cruciate-deficient knee. Part I: the long-term functional disability in athletically active individuals. J Bone Joint Surg 1983;65A:154–162.

Ohkoshi Y, Ohkoshi M, Nagasaki S, Ono A, Hashimoto T, Yamane S. The effect of cryotherapy on intraarticular temperature and postoperative care after anterior cruciate ligament reconstruction. Am J Sports Med 1999;27(3):357–362.

O'Neill DB. Arthroscopically assisted reconstruction of the anterior cruciate ligament. A prospective randomized analysis of three techniques. J Bone Joint Surg Am 1996;78(6):806–813.

Palmer I. On injuries to the knee joint. A clinical study. Acta Orthop Scand 1938;81(Suppl 53).

Paulos LE, Cherf J, Rosenberg TD. Anterior cruciate ligament reconstruction with autografts. Clin Sports Med 1991;10:469–485.

Pavlovich R. High-frequency electrical cautery stimulation in the treatment of displaced meniscal tears. Arthroscopy 1998;14:566–571.

Pressman A, Johnson DH. ACL reconstruction with BioScrews and semi-tendinosus: 2 year results. In: Arthroscopy Association of North America Annual Meeting, 2001. Seattle, WA.

Rosaeg OP, Krepski B, Cicutti N, et al. Effect of pre-emptive multi-modal analgesia for arthroscopic knee ligament repair. Regional Anesth Pain Med 2001; 26:125–130.

Rosenberg TD, et al. Arthroscopic meniscal repair evaluated with repeat arthroscopy. Arthroscopy 1986;2:14–21.

Shelbourne KD, Patel DV, McCarroll JR. Management of anterior cruciate ligament injuries in skeletally immature adolescents. Knee Surg Sports Traumatol Arthrosc 1996;4(2):68–74.

Shelbourne KD, Davis TJ, Klootwyk TE. Correlation of the intercondylar notch width of the femur to the width of the anterior and posterior cruciate ligaments. Knee Surg Sports Traumatol Arthrosc 1999;7:209–214.

Shelbourne, KD, JG. Patient Selection for Anterior Cruciate Ligament Reconstruction. Operative Techniques in Sports Medicine, 1993;1(7):16–21.

Shelbourne KD, Johnson GE. Locked bucket-handle meniscal tears in knees with chronic anterior cruciate ligament deficiency. Am J Sports Med 1993; 21(6):779–782.

Shelbourne KD, McCarroll JR, Patell DV. Anterior cruciate ligament reconstruction in athletes with an ossicle with Osgoode-Schlatters disease. Arthroscopy 1996;12(5):556–560.

Shelbourne KD, Patell DV. Timing of surgery in anterior cruciate ligament-injured knees. Knee Surg Sports Traumatol Arthrosc 1995;3:148–156.

Shelbourne KD, Paul AN. Accelerated rehabilitation after anterior cruciate ligament reconstruction. Am J Sports Med 1990;18:292–299.

Siddles JA, Larson RV, Garbini JL, et al. Ligament length relationships in the moving knee. J Orthop Res 1988;6:593–610.

Simonian PT, Metcalf MH, Larson RV. Anterior cruciate ligament injuries in the skeletally immature patient. Am J Orthop 1999;28(11):624–628.

Stadelmaier DM, Arnoczky SP, Dodds J, et al. The effect of drilling and soft tissue grafting across open growth plates. A histologic study. Am J Sports Med 1995;23:431–435.

Staubli HU, Schatzmann L, Brunner P, Rincon L, Nolte LP. Mechanical tensile properties of the quadriceps tendon and patellar ligament in young adults. Am J Sports Med 1999;27(1):27–34.

Traina SM, Bromberg DF. ACL injury patterns in women. Orthopedics 1997; 20:545–549, 550–551.

Viola RVR. Intra-articular ACL reconstruction in the over-40-year-old patient. Knee Surg Sports Traumatol Arthroscopy 1999;7(1):25–28.

Weiler A, Richter M, Schmidmaier G, Kandziora F, Sudkamp NP. The Endo-pearl device increases fixation strength and eliminates construct slippage of hamstring tendon grafts with interference screw fixation. Arthroscopy 2001;17(4):353–359.

Yu WD, Panossian V, Hatch JD, Liu SH, Finerman GA. Combined effects of estrogen and progesterone on the anterior cruciate ligament. Clin Orthop 2001;383:268–281.

Yunes M, Richmond JC, Engels EA, Pinczewski LA. Patellar versus hamstring tendons in anterior cruciate ligament reconstruction: A meta-analysis. Arthroscopy 2001;17(3):248–257.

Zhang A, Arnold JA, Williams T, et al. Repairs by trephination and suturing of longitudinal injuries in the avascular area of the meniscus in goats. Am J Sports Med 1995;23:35–41.

Index